Neuroanatomy
and Cranial
Computed Tomography

Neuroanatomy and Cranial Computed Tomography

By Hans-Joachim Kretschmann and Wolfgang Weinrich

Foreword by Ruth G. Ramsey
Drawings by Rudolf Mutschall
225 Mostly Colored Illustrations

1986
Georg Thieme Verlag Stuttgart · New York
Thieme Inc. New York

Prof. Dr. med. Hans-Joachim KRETSCHMANN
Chairman of Department of Neuroanatomy
Hannover Medical School
Konstanty-Gutschow-Str. 8, D-3000 Hannover 61
West Germany

Prof. Dr. med. Wolfgang WEINRICH
Chairman of Neurological Clinic
Krankenhaus Nordstadt
Haltenhoffstr. 41, D-3000 Hannover 1
West Germany

Dentist Rudolf MUTSCHALL
Department of Neuroanatomy
Hannover Medical School
Konstanty-Gutschow-Str. 8, D-3000 Hannover 61
West Germany

Library of Congress Cataloging-in-Publication Data

Kretschmann, Hans Joachim.
Neuroanatomy and cranial computed tomography.
Translation of: Neuroanatomie der kraniellen Computertomographie.
Bibliography: p. includes index.
1. Brain–Anatomy–Atlases. 2. Brain–Radiography––Atlases. 3. Skull–Anatomy–Atlases. 4. Skull–Radiography–Atlases. 5. Tomography–Atlases.
6. Neuroanatomy–Atlases. I. Weinrich, Wolfgang.
II. Title. [DNLM: 1. Brain–pathology–atlases.
2. Brain–radiography–Atlases. 3. Tomography,
X-Ray Computed–atlases. WL 17 K915n]
QM455.K69513   1986   611.81'0222   85-24674

© 1986, Georg Thieme Verlag, P. O. Box 732, D-7000 Stuttgart 1, FRG
Typesetting: Kittelberger, Reutlingen
(Linotron 202, System 5)
Printed in Germany by Grammlich, Pliezhausen

ISBN 3-13-672601-4 (Thieme Verlag, Stuttgart)
ISBN 0-86577-212-6 (Thieme Inc., New York)
1 2 3 4 5

Foreword

The authors have reviewed in detail the normal neuroanatomic features that are identified on standard computed tomograms. The illustrations are clear and well demarcated. The authors have elected to use line drawings and tracings from the actual CT scans rather than using the scans themselves. This in no way detracts from the information available. In fact, this technique makes the normal anatomy more easily identifiable. In those anatomic areas, where certain functional neuroanatomic pathways are of clinical importance, the authors elected to embellish the illustrations with the appropriate microscopic fiber tracts even though they are not visible on the CT scans. This allows students of CT as well as students of the neurosciences to appreciate the exact anatomic location of these important neurological structures without requiring the use of a neuroanatomy book. The angles used for the CT scans are those which are very familiar to those who use CT scans routinely.

There is an extensive discussion of the neuroanatomy of a variety of common neurologic diseases and syndromes that can be identified through clinical examination and CT examination. The review of neuroanatomy is extensive and useful and serves to enhance the understanding of the appearance of the CT scans. The pathways are discussed and illustrated in a very practical way without obscuring the stated purpose of the book, which is to illustrate the normal neurofunctional and neuroanatomic CT appearence. This allows all students of the neurosciences to become familiar with these classical disease entities without being overcome by minutae. Those in radiology and neuroradiology can readily understand the presentation of these clinical diseases and syndromes and appreciate the correlation with the CT scan. Those students and practitioners in the other neurosciences such as neurosurgery, neurology, neuropediatrics, as well as medical students can appreciate the correlation with the CT scans.

The discussion of the workings of the CT scanner, discussion of magnetic resonance and excellent drawings and correlation with the anatomic structures make this a valuable text, that can be used on a daily basis for clinical evaluation and correlation with the anticipated anatomic location of the abnormality. In addition to the review of the various pathways of the neuroanatomic structures, there are review and discussions of CSF dynamics, the basal cisterns, and relationships of the structures at the skull base with the intracranial contents. The book provides good guidelines regarding the use of external landmarks for intracranial localization.

It is a pleasure to recommend this book as a welcome and very practical text-atlas for use on a daily basis. It can be used not just for correlation with the CT scans but in a very practical way for the evaluation of the patient with neurologic disease. I believe that the reader will find this book just as helpful for evaluation of the neurologic disease as for the CT findings. The radiologist will enjoy the practical, no nonsense approach to neuropathology and disease topography and will be better equipped to relate the neuropathology and topography to her or his clinical colleagues while the clinicians will easily understand the anatomic illustrations.

The entire atlas is straightforward and understandable. The illustrations are clear and well chosen. It is obvious that the authors are very familiar with their subject and are able to impart this knowledge to their readers. The users of this book will find it a practical and welcome addition to their medical library.

Ruth G. Ramsey, M.D. Chicago, Ill.

Preface

Cranial computed tomography marks a great advance in neurological medicine: brain parts and brain structures can be visualized which could be viewed only at the operating and/or sectioning table thirteen years ago. Today a neurosurgeon generally needs CT images to plan the best surgical strategy. Just to give one example, with the help of computed tomography brain tumors can be diagnosed with a probability of 95% (Kazner, Wende, Grumme, Lanksch, and Stochdorph, 1981). The magnetic resonance (MR) imaging, as a new computer imaging technique, promises to bring about a "small revolution for medicine" (Habermehl and Graul, 1982).

These computer techniques produce images of planes which need for their interpretation by the user a three-dimensional concept of brain structures. Spatial knowledge of the neurofunctional systems makes possible the prediction of neurological deficits from the location of the lesion. Therefore, in this book the main pathways of the neurofunctional systems are demonstrated in the customary CT planes. Furthermore, cerebral vessels and their territories are illustrated and described according to their clinical relevance, as arteries are diseased frequently and angiographies have to be correlated with CT images.

The illustrations and the text are meant to be a day-to-day tool for the clinician. The book is intended for Neurologists, Neurosurgeons, Neuropediatricians, Neuroradiologists, Radiologists, Neurophysiologists, Neuropathologists, as well as physicians in Internal Medicine, Traumatologists, Oncologists, and students and physicians interested in the neurosciences. For the illustrations a new drawing technique was developed: the anatomical structures are illustrated in gray values which correlate with those of the CT images.

In the text an anglicized international anatomical nomenclature is used, as large international bibliographies (Index Medicus, National Library of Medicine Washington, D.C.), word processing programs like the international classification of diseases, injuries, and causes of death (SNOMED and ICD), as well as recommendations of the World Health Organization are based on this Anglo-American terminology. Important clinical expressions that differ from the international nomenclature are mentioned in the text and illustrations.

The English edition has been expanded by a chapter about the arterial territories of the brain in axial sections. Thirteen new illustrations have been added, and the references have been brought up to date. Some parts of the text were extended to take account of the comments of critical readers of the German edition.

Hans-Joachim Kretschmann   Wolfgang Weinrich

Acknowledgements

This book was made possible through the help of many colleagues, co-workers, and others. We are grateful for their support. Their part in the completion of the book cannot easily be given in an order of precedence. Therefore, we want to express our gratitude in the order of the development of this project.

We were encouraged by Prof. Dr. med. Helmut Künkel, Prof. Dr. med. Parviz Mehraein, Prof. Dr. med. Hans Schliack, Hannover Medical School, Prof. Dr. med. Hans-Joachim Löblich, Krankenhaus Nordstadt, Hannover, and Prof. Dr. med. et. Dipl. Math. Friedrich Wingert, Institute for Medical Informatics and Biomathematics, University of Münster, to start this project. Many suggestions and ideas originated during three scientific stays at the Yakovlev Collection in Washington, D.C., which were supported by the Deutsche Forschungsgemeinschaft (Kr 289/11-14) and the National Institute of Neurological and Communicative Disorders and Stroke (NINCDS). We are especially indepted to Dr. Paul I. Yakovlev†. For the graphic illustrations of the blood vessels and the neurofunctional systems the publications by Huber, Krayenbühl, Yasargil (1982) and by Nieuwenhuys, Voogd, Huijzen (1981) were important guidelines.

Dr. med. h.c. Günther Hauff, Thieme Verlag Stuttgart, made available the usage of modern printing methods. His associates Mr. Rainer Zepf recommended the Ulano technique for production of the illustrations and Mr. Gert Krüger was responsible for the excellent technique of printing.

Dentist Rudolf Mutschall developed a new drawing technique with gray values, which give an impression of the anatomical sections similar to those of CT images. Dentist Marianne Prien was involved in developing the drawings, in the identification and labelling of the cerebral vessels and in preparing the print copies. The photos and the complete technical processing of the head sections were executed by Mr. Karl Rust. Due to his masterly skill the project has a solid technical background. Mr. Karl Rust and Mr. Klaus-Martin Podzuweit built a styrofoam model of the forebrain. Mrs. Imola Braun assisted in the drawing of the foils.

The histological work was done by Mrs. Heike Fahlbusch, Mrs. Erika Sterner, Mrs. Gisela Wiese, and Mr. Klaus-Martin Podzuweit. The X-rays were taken by Mrs. Helga Fehse, Krankenhaus Nordstadt, Hannover, Mr. Wilfried Fischer, and Prof. Dr. med. vet. Werner Küpper, Department of Experimental Animals, (Director: Prof. Dr. med. vet. Klaus Gärtner) Hannover Medical School. For the MR images of the head, as an example of a new imaging technique, we owe thanks to Prof. Dr. med. Heinz Hundeshagen, Head of the Department of Nuclear Medicine and Biophysics, Hannover Medical School. After completion of the German manuscript we were advised by Dr. med. Gerhard Bierling, Radiologist, Hannover, Prof. Dr. med. Rolf Hassler†, and Dr. rer. nat. Heinz Stephan, Max-Planck-Institute for Brain Research, Frankfurt/Main, Dr. med. Hans-Jürgen Keller, Radiologist, Helmstedt, Prof. Dr. med. Hans-Jürgen Kuhn, Director, Institute of Anatomy, University of Göttingen, Prof. Dr. med. Helmut Künkel, Head of the Department of Neurology and Clinical Neurophysiology, Hannover Medical School, Prof. Dr. med. Dieter Seitz, Head of the Department of Neurology, General Hospital St. Georg, Hamburg, Prof. Dr. med. Wolfhard Winkelmüller, Department of Neurosurgery, Paracelsus Klinik, Osnabrück. Their suggestions were included in the text and the illustrations. We appreciate the proofreading by physician Eckhard Faber, cand. med. Michael Gerke, and Mrs. Frauke Weinrich.

In our search for references we were aided by Mrs. Erika Battermann and Mrs. Inge-Lore Wunderer. The manuscript was typed with great precision by Mrs. Waltraud Reichert. Helpful were word processing programs by Dipl. Math. Andreas Herrmann, sort programs by cand. rer. nat. Gerd Fleischer, and the insertion of type setting codes by cand. rer. nat. Frank Mittendorf.

The English translation developed through several stages: cand. med. vet. Thomas Geimer translated the first draft. In further improvements participated: cand. med. et phil. Susanne Kretschmann, physician Angela Krönauer, Mrs. Susan Mary Mullarki, physician Frank Dressler, cand. med. Wolfrid T. Lübke, cand. med. Axel Piepgras, Dr. med. Claudia Rüffer, Dr. med. Gisela Rilling, Prof. Dr. Keki Turel, Bombay, India. The responsibility for the translation rests with one author (K.).

After completion of the manuscript we are grateful for comments of Marjorie LeMay, M.D., Professor of Radiology, Harvard University Health Services Cambridge, Mass., Ruth G. Ramsey, M.D., Professor of Radiology, Rush Presbyterian St. Luke's Medical Center, Chicago, Ill., and M.J.T. FitzGerald, M.D., Professor of Anatomy, Chairman of Department of Anatomy, Galway, Ireland (author of the helpful book Neuroanatomy Basic and Applied, published by Baillière Tindall in 1985).

We want to express our appreciation and gratitude to all those who made possible the production of this book.

Hans-Joachim Kretschmann   Wolfgang Weinrich

Contents

1 Introduction

1.1 Background and Objectives

The year 1972 marked the development of the computed tomographic scanner by Hounsfield. Later that year, Ambrose (5) incorporated computed tomography (CT) in the diagnosis of brain diseases. The advantages of this new technique for medicine are evident. During the past decade CT scanners have been improved and more recently magnetic resonance imaging (MR) has opened up new diagnostic possibilities (3, 20, 29, 60, 61, 83, 89, 92, 182, 218, 252, 315, 326).

Computed tomography produces cross-sectional images of the human head as seen at various angles perpendicular to the longitudinal axis of the body. Compared with the images obtained in "classical" neuroanatomy CT analysis produces unconventional views of the human brain for the following reasons: during human evolution, the forebrain moved from its original in-line horizontal location with the brain stem to an obtuse angle of 110°–120°. This relocation was caused by the development of an upright posture and an enormous increase in size of the neocortex, which displaced the phylogenetically old cortical structures of the forebrain. In most textbooks of neuroanatomy the human brain is illustrated using at least two cross-sectional series. One transverse series is cut perpendicularly to the longitudinal axis of the forebrain (Forel's axis), the other transverse series is cut perpendicularly to the longitudinal axis of the brain stem (Meynert's axis). This procedure facilitates extrapolation of neuroanatomical results to the human brain originally derived from animals. In most mammals the axes of the forebrain and brain stem are nearly the same, whereas in the human brain an obtuse angle is formed.

CT sections in humans are made at different angles to the "classical" ones and do not allow for such a comparison. One plane alone cannot produce images of both the human forebrain and the brain stem, which correspond with those images taken from conventional neuroanatomical sections. There is, therefore, no "ideal" CT imaging plane for the axial sections of the human brain.

Ambrose (5) chose the canthomeatal plane as the most appropriate imaging plane for CT scans. Running from the lateral corner of the eyelid (canthus) to the external acoustic meatus, Ambrose (5) named it the orbitomeatal plane. The features and advantages of this and other cross-sectional planes will be discussed in Chapter 1.4 . CT scans of the head made parallel to the canthomeatal plane differ significantly from conventional neuroanatomical images. CT may be used to best advantage only if the investigator has sufficient knowledge of three-dimensional structures to be able to interpret such unconventional images. Up to now, medical students have seldom been trained in the interpretation of neuroanatomical structures as seen in CT sections. As a result, numerous books have been published during the past decade that demonstrate the gross neuroanatomy of the head using axial sections (25, 43, 81, 91, 97, 145, 149, 153, 168, 171, 183, 188, 189, 192, 199, 204, 258, 297, 299, 309).

Neurofunctional systems, however, cannot be described by gross anatomy alone. Specific neuronal tracts, for example, often remain inconspicuous in histological preparations. Only a synopsis of findings taken from macroscopic, microscopic, embryologic, neuropathologic, and comparative studies permits a reliable illustration of human neurofunctional systems.

The objectives of this book are as follows:

1. The main tracts of the neurofunctional systems will be presented in axial sections as clearly as possible. The brain is oriented in a rectangular coordinate system and sectioned in serial slices at distances of one centimeter. Each slice is drawn to scale on a gray background as seen in the canthomeatal parallel plane from above. The series of illustrations are generally presented in groups of four per page. These images are arranged from left to right down the page as taken from the sectional series. The reader will be able to mentally construct a three-dimensional representation of the brain structures (Figs. 5–18) and the neurofunctional systems (Figs. 42–64) by superimposing the individual illustrations of the series correctly. The head is visualized in a x, y, z coordinate system. The x and y axes are the top and side edges, respectively, of each illustration. Vertical to the section plane is the z axis.

2. Three-dimensional topographical reproductions of neurofunctional pathways (Figs. 42–64) aid in deducing monosymptomatic or polysymptomatic disorders from the location of the lesions. With this in mind, we have included descriptions of both the clinically important neurofunctional systems and the symptoms resulting from lesions. The topography of lesions in axial sections together with knowledge of spatial relationships can help to account for neurofunctional deficits.

3. Pathological changes in cerebral blood vessels are a major cause of brain diseases. Consequently, detailed attention is given to the blood vessels and their territories in the cross-sectional brain slices. Furthermore, these slices are compared with corresponding angiographic images. In this manner, we hope to facilitate not only the interpretation of angiocomputed tomography but also the comparison of computed tomographic and angiographic findings.

4. A new drawing technique has been developed, which produces more exact illustrations of the corresponding CT scans than previously described methods. The anatomical structures illustrated are shown in various shades of gray corresponding to those in CT scans. All drawings in the atlas section of this book are delineated from original sections (Chap. 1.3). Some structures, that are only detectable microscopically, such as cortical areas or specific pathways, were added to the illustrations.

5. The graphic representation of the neurofunctional systems in the cross sections should provide a basis for new image processing techniques such as positron emission tomography or magnetic resonance (MR) imaging. Such imaging techniques can further increase the diagnostic value of computed tomography (Chaps. 2.2 and 2.4). With the exception of four exemplary CT scans (Figs. 40a–d) a systematic comparison of CT images with the actual anatomical sections is not included.

6. Neuroanatomical structures and their variations, that are of obvious clinical relevance, are elaborated in the text section of this book. Anatomical details of purely systematic, embryological, comparative, and microscopical interest are described briefly in Chapters 1.5 and 5. Numbers given in parentheses refer to publications specifically relevant to the discussed topic.

This book is intended to be used as a day-to-day tool in clinical work by neurologists, neurosurgeons, neuropediatricians, neuroradiologists, neurophysiologists, as well as by doctors of internal medicine, traumatologists, otolaryngologists, and oncologists. It will also be useful for those students and physicians interested in neural science. This book presents the main neurofunctional systems and relevant structures in axial sections. As a diagnostic tool it facilitates the interpretation of the various modern imaging processing techniques developed for the head by providing the necessary neurotopographic and neurofunctional orientation. In addition, it allows a critical correlation between clinical symptoms and pathological CT findings. Speculative information and unconfirmed scientific research has not been included.

1.2 Postmortem and Histological Changes of the Brain Structures

Postmortem and histological changes in the brain must be taken into consideration when findings of anatomical dissections are transferred to living patients. Under in vivo and postmortem conditions accurate determination of blood, cerebrospinal fluid, and brain tissue volumes in the respective compartments of the cranial cavity is difficult. Some investigations provide evidence of a partial diffusion of cerebrospinal fluid into the brain tissue after death. Following death, the average volume of cerebrospinal compartments decreases. In 159 examined cases the volume of cerebrospinal fluid averaged 100 ml 3 hours post mortem and only 49 ml after 21 hours (273).

The difference between the volume of the cranial cavity and the brain decreases after death (216). The postmortem brain volume increases as cerebrospinal fluid is absorbed: the degree of absorption depends on the time interval between death and autopsy. Assuming an average of 100–150 ml cerebrospinal fluid and 1200–1400 ml brain volume in living adults, an error of 5% can be expected after half of the cerebrospinal fluid has steadily diffused into the brain tissue following death. This diffusion is likely to be non-linear in nature. The postmortem volume increase in more heavily affected brain areas will be correspondingly higher. Because the CSF is absorbed postmortem, a correlation of the size of cisterns found at the autopsy with in vivo conditions may only be made with caution.

An apparent change in the relative proportion and position of the brain stem to the forebrain is usually observed in brains fixed outside the cranial cavity. In most cases, the brain is suspended by the basilar artery during fixation. Because the specific gravity of the brain is slightly higher than that of the formalin fixative, the forebrain, which hangs downward in the fixation solution, sinks. With its occipital pole sinking first, the forebrain alters its proportion and position relative to the brain stem. As a result, intracerebral proportions of brains fixed outside the cranial cavity differ significantly from those in vivo. Consequently, for anatomic comparisons with CT images it is necessary to use brains fixed inside the cranial cavity rather than those fixed outside.

When embedded in paraffin or celloidin for histological preparations, the brain loses 40–50% of its volume (108, 157). Two types of brain tissue, however, do not shrink equally in paraffin embedded preparations: gray matter, due to its higher water content, shrinks more than white matter (158). 84% of the volume of the frontal cortex and 71% of the volume of the white matter are water. During the embedding procedure the frontal cortex loses 51% and the white matter about 42% of its volume (158). Findings concerning size and form of brain structures taken from histological preparations, therefore, can be correlated only approximately with in vivo conditions.

Thus, it is quite obvious that postmortem factors can alter the relative position of brain structures. Nevertheless, the results of stereotactic operations support the assumption that the location of in vivo brain structures can be estimated from anatomical sections if the factors causing interference are taken into account. Prior to stereotactic operations, the positions of brain structures relative to the bicommissural plane (Chap. 1.4) or to the base line between the interventricular foramen and the posterior commissure, are calculated to the nearest millimeter (105, 264, 265, 266). To date, for most neurofunctional systems there have been no clinical requirements to conduct such calculations.

1.3 Material and Methods

After extensive deliberation we selected the head of a 44-year-old male (H 22/77) from the collection of human dissection material at the Department of Anatomy, Hannover Medical School, Hannover, West Germany. The deceased was 176 cm tall and weighed approximately 80 kg. The head was relatively large, measuring 17.1 cm at the widest point above the external acoustic meatus and 23.4 cm at the longest span between the glabella and the opisthion. The width-length index was calculated at 73%. The facial height was 12.5 cm measured between the nasion and the gnathion. The greatest distance between the two most lateral points of the zygomatic bones was 16.6 cm. The face index was calculated at 75%. The cause of death was suicide by hanging.

Cerebrospinal fluid was extracted by suboccipital and lumbar puncture from the cadaver and was replaced by an equal amount of a 37% formalin Merck-solution slowly injected into the subarachnoid space. Perfusion was carried out through the femoral arteries with a fixative containing 86 parts 96% alcohol, 8 parts 37% formalin, 3 parts glycerine DAB 7, and 3 parts of a saturated phenol DAB 8 solution (all parts given in parts of volume). After taking posterior-anterior and lateral X-rays, the head was examined with an EMI CT scan No. 1010 in seven double sections parallel to the canthomeatal plane. Four CT images taken from this series are reproduced in Figures 40a–d. Air is present in the subarachnoid space. It should be noted that postmortem changes and fixation reduced the density-contrast of the brain tissue.

The head was stored at –26°C for six days. It was sectioned along the canthomeatal plane using a band-saw KS 400, made by Reich, Nürtingen, West Germany. One centimeter thick slices were removed in sequence using a special adjustment guide. The thickness of each slice was reduced by 1 mm due to the cutting-width of the band-saw blade. Two deep cuts through the skin were made perpendicularly to the canthomeatal plane in the median plane and in plane A around the head. Plane A is located just in front of the ear running perpendicularly to the median and canthomeatal planes. These circular cuts served in each slice as markers for the median plane and plane A. The canthomeatal plane, median plane, and plane A correspond to the x, y, z cartesian coordinates, and thereby provide a three-dimensional orientation. The cross-sectional surfaces of the slices were photographed and reproduced on a scale of 1:1. The photographs were traced in ink on transparent plastic overlays. To maximize accuracy, the illustrations were compared throughout this process with the original slices. The smaller structures were identified under a Zeiss stereomicroscope using an improved light source (Volpi halogen cold mercury lamp Intralux 150 H) (6). Gennari's band in the visual cortex, corona radiata, and alveus of the hippocampus were distinctly visible on these alcohol-formalin fixed brain slices. Small arteries were histologically differentiated from veins of similar size. The slices were compared with neurohistological sections from the collection of the Department of Neuroanatomy at Hannover Medical School. Serial sections of another brain (H 22/81) of a 51-year-old male cut parallel to the canthomeatal plane were particularly helpful.

To aid the identification of the various sulci and gyri, a 1:1 styrofoam model of the above mentioned brain H 22/77 was built and compared with macroscopical sections of other brains.

Towards the final phase of our examination we assembled the individual slices. A lateral X-ray was taken to determine the exact location of the sectioning plane through the head. To compensate for the 1 mm loss in thickness of the slices due to the width of the blade (14 cuts account for 14 mm), the X-ray was cut into strips and remounted with a 1 mm space between the individual slice. Figure 2 shows the final result. The medial and lateral views of the brain (Figs. 3 and 4) were assembled with slices cut from the right hemisphere and the right half of the brain stem. The hemisphere itself, however, had to be reconstructed first. This was accomplished by a midline cut through the cross sections and by assembling the resulting individually freed halves into a complete hemisphere and brain stem. These slices were photographed. Corrections were made for the corresponding 1 mm intervals as mentioned above. The lateral view of the ventricular system (Fig. 26) was graphically reconstructed from the canthomeatal plane using a Wang 2200 computer (program by Dr. B. Sauer) and topographically superimposed on the X-ray image of the head (Fig. 2).

The section or slice number is indicated by a circle in Figures 1a, 2, 3, 4, 26, and in the serial illustrations. The small cranial arteries, which lie between the sulci of the cerebrum, are often highly convoluted and branched. Exact reconstruction of the course of these fine arteries on the 1 cm thick slices was not possible in all regions. With the precuneal artery, for instance, it was impossible to differentiate between the superior and inferior precuneal arteries. General reference to the precuneal artery must therefore suffice (Figs. 15a.13, 16a.8, 17a.8). Similarly, branches of the parietal and temporal arteries of the middle cerebral artery are not subdivided further (Figs. 13a.17, 14a.11, 15a.12, 9a.8, 10a.8, 11a.10). Small arteries, such as the lateral frontobasal artery, which run totally within a slice parallel to the sectioning plane, are not cut and consequently are not shown in the illustrations.

The head of the 44-year-old male, from which the drawings in the atlas (Figs. 5–18), the X-rays (Figs. 19–24) and the CT scans (Figs. 40a–d) were made, shows some anatomical peculiarities. The paranasal sinuses are extremely large, the sphenoid sinus in particular (Figs. 7a.7 and 8a.8). The pineal gland is exceptionally small (Fig. 12a.18). The veins are enlarged due to strangulation. Brain edema is slight. The ventricles are narrow. These morphological features are clearly seen in the illustrations.

1.4 Axial Section Planes

The horizontal plane through the upright human body is called the transverse plane. Clinically speaking, a plane lying at a slight inclination to a transverse plane is called an axial plane. Because of frequent deviations of the vertebral column, anthropologists and clinicians have established the following cranial points of reference for the respective sectioning planes:

Reid's base line or "Deutsche Horizontale" (abbreviated DH) extends from the lower orbital margin to the upper edge of the external acoustic (auditory) meatus (Fig. 1a, DH).

The canthomeatal plane connects the lateral angle of the eye (lateral canthus) with the center of the external acoustic meatus. Ambrose (5) called it the orbitomeatal plane. This term, however, is also used as a synonym for the horizontal plane (153, 297). In order to avoid ambiguity, the expression canthomeatal plane is preferred.

Radiologists, furthermore, refer to the infraorbitomeatal plane. The infraorbitomeatal plane is inclined approximately 15° towards the canthomeatal plane (258) and runs through the lower orbital margin and the center of the external acoustic meatus. The supraorbitomeatal plane passes through the

upper margin of the orbit and the center of the external acoustic meatus (258).

For clinical CT examination of the brain the parallel canthomeatal planes are generally used. A complete cranial examination in this plane requires fewer slices of uniform thickness than choosing perfectly horizontal planes. This is accounted for by the flattened external form of the human brain and the location of the natural longitudinal axis through the brain. This axis runs more parallel to the canthomeatal plane than to the horizontal plane (Figs. 3 and 4, DH). Consequently, by using a sectioning plane parallel to the canthomeatal plane, the relative time of examination is shortened and the patient's total radiation dose is reduced. Furthermore, since X-ray technicians can easily identify the canthomeatal plane, the procedure is easy to repeat. From a theoretical point of view, the choice of the canthomeatal plane is supported by the parallel location of the bicommissural line on a statistical average. The bicommissural line connects the superior margin of the anterior commissure with the inferior margin of the posterior commissure (296). The bicommissural line is an important orientation guide in stereotactic operations and, likewise, a suitable natural reference for neuroanatomic comparisons. In a sample of 50 brains, the angle between the canthomeatal plane and the bicommissural line revealed less than a 2° difference on the average. In two cases differences of 9° and –5° (standard deviation = 1.4) were observed (296). The inherent variability of individual brain structures, when examined in one of the extracerebral reference systems, is greater than using one based on the bicommissural line or similar intracerebral coordinates (21, 148, 198).

As already mentioned in Chapter 1.1, there is no ideal sectioning plane for cranial CT scans. Planes other than the canthomeatal plane may be required for diverse clinical examinations. Sections parallel to the infraorbitomeatal plane, for instance, are suitable for an examination of the orbit and its contents. As a rule, the optic nerve runs parallel to this plane. In addition, the external muscles of the eyes can be visualized clearly. In sectioning planes parallel to the infraorbitomeatal plane at supraventricular levels, the central gyrus with the neighboring precentral and postcentral gyri is located farther dorsal than in the canthomeatal parallel planes (258).

Sections made parallel to the supraorbitomeatal plane are especially useful when examining structures in the posterior cranial fossa. In the supraventricular slices the central sulcus and adjacent structures appear to lie in a more ventral position than in the canthomeatal parallel planes (258). The canthomeatal parallel planes shown in Figures 1a, 2, 3, and 4 illustrate the altered appearance of the sections after a flexion or an extension of the head. A standardized sectioning plane, which permits a direct

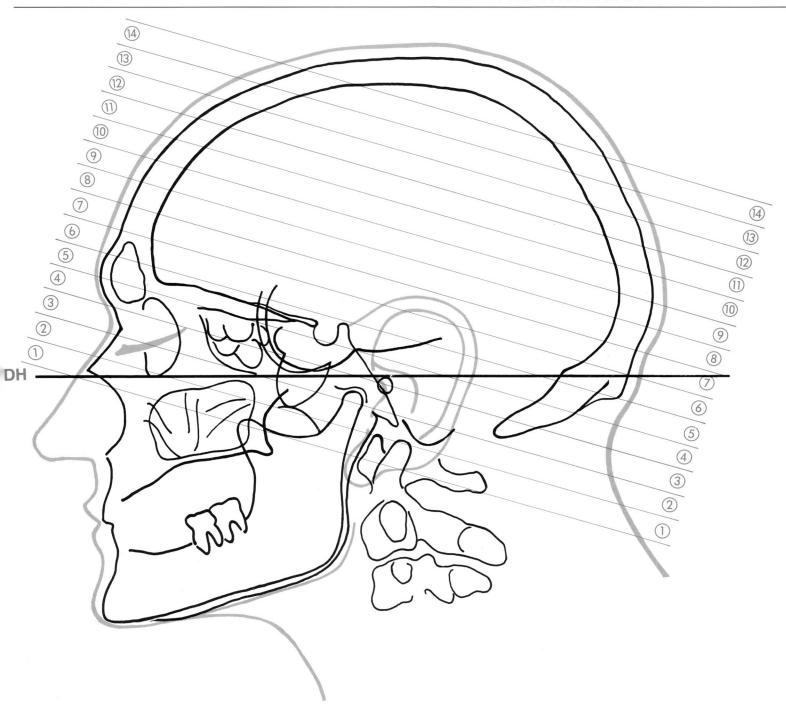

Fig. 1a Canthomeatal parallel planes are shown on the lateral surface of the head of a 44-year-old male. The 14 slices are described in a caudal to cranial order in the atlas portion of this book (Figs. 5–18). The encircled numbers indicate the numbers of 1 cm thick slices, which are illustrated in the atlas as seen from above. The illustrated surface of each section, therefore, represents the line above the encircled number of the corresponding slice.

DH = Reid's base line = "Deutsche Horizontale".

comparison of CT scans of different patients, is the basic requirement for routine CT examinations. The previous discussion shows that the canthomeatal plane is well suited for this purpose.

1.5 Terminology and References

The international anatomical nomenclature serves a better understanding between the various nations of the world. For this reason, we decided to use an Anglicized version of the international anatomical nomenclature (71, 130), even though such technical terms have a number of problems of their own. Without doubt, the addition of new anatomical terms to this nomenclature is essential. The existing Mexico City nomenclature names only 5600 anatomical structures of the great number known. In the era of angiography, for instance, it became necessary for commissions to name branches of the main cerebral arteries which had not been listed earlier. International agreements generally conflict with national conventions. With this in mind, we have included – enclosed in parentheses – the clinically used synonyms in the illustrations and in the text at least after the first mention of an international anatomical name. These more common names also appear in the index.

The international anatomical nomenclature differentiates between arteria and ramus. Frequently, the diameters of these so-called rami are greater than those of the arteries themselves, e.g., ramus parieto-occipitalis and anterolateral central arteries. The term ramus is also applied to veins, nerves, bones, and bronchial branches. Therefore, in accordance with the more common clinical usage, we will refer to all arterial branches by the less ambiguous term artery (128, 257, 296, 310).

Numbers in parentheses refer to publications listed in the bibliography (see Chap. 5):

General neuroanatomy: (9, 13, 33, 41, 48, 54, 72, 74, 76, 88, 113, 138, 139, 140, 153, 161, 162, 167, 168, 177, 181, 187, 206, 207, 223, 228, 243, 263, 265, 276, 277, 279, 283, 300, 318, 319)

Neuroanatomic techniques: (108, 114, 118)

Neuroembryology: (8, 95, 172, 278, 286)

Neurohistology: (37, 64, 224, 332)

Comparative neuroanatomy: (285, 287)

Special neuroanatomy; brain stem: (117, 213, 245, 284)

Cerebellum: (7, 63, 136, 215, 248)

Diencephalon: (38, 58, 59, 103, 104, 105, 107, 179, 195, 203, 212, 311, 312)

Telencephalon: (28, 42, 111, 150, 289, 331)

Neurology: (1, 26, 34, 39, 55, 62, 82, 124, 196, 197, 219, 229, 230, 256, 267, 301)

Neuroradiology: (44, 47, 65, 81, 91, 96, 97, 128, 144, 175, 183, 184, 188, 189, 199, 205, 226, 237, 238, 240, 241, 247, 257, 258, 272, 296, 297, 298, 302, 309, 313)

1.6 Notes for the Reader

As a rule, computed tomographic examinations of the brain start at the base. CT images are evaluated together with the neighboring images from the sequence. With these two factors in mind, we have arranged our descriptions of the anatomic sections in the corresponding sequence, i.e., Figures 1a, 2, 3, and 4. Only the cranial views of the anatomical sections are shown in Figures 5–18. The left side of the body is consistently represented as the left side of the illustrations.

In the illustrations the anatomical structures are labelled with numbers. When possible, these numbers were placed in the optic center of the structure. Where this was graphically impossible, an indicating line was added. The numbers are arranged continuously from left to right and from top to bottom, corresponding with the normal reading sequence of the Western reader. In areas with a high density of numbers neighboring structures are numbered continuously without regard to their arrangement from left to right and top to bottom. Paired structures, which appear symmetrically, are labelled once only. Paired structures, which appear in different positions in the two hemispheres of the brain, are labelled twice with the same number. Structures, that are cut more than once in the same sectioning plane, such as the superior sagittal sinus (Fig. 17a.2), maintain their number throughout the illustration (in this case twice). Each illustration is numbered independently. The insula, which appears in some illustrations, is listed in the index under Figures F11b.9, F12b.13, F13b.14, etc. The numbering scheme used for blood vessels (Figs. 28–33) takes into account both regions and direction of flow. As far as the neurofunctional systems are concerned, individual structures are labelled throughout the sequence of the illustrations.

2 Computed Tomography and CT Guideline Structures

The high density resolution of CT makes possible, for the first time, in vivo identification of macroscopic cranial structures and partial differentiation of gray and white matter despite the fact that the brain is enclosed in an X-ray dense skull. According to Hounsfield, CT provides a density resolution nearly 100 times more sensitive than that of conventional X-ray techniques (125). Because of low resolution, the latter fail to detect the relatively small differences in the densities of the soft brain tissues (211). As a result, the cranial cavity appears empty in conventional X-rays. In order to indirectly delineate intracranial brain structures using conventional neuroradiological techniques, a contrast medium has to be utilized. Two such techniques are pneumoencephalography and angiography (199, 200).

Interpretation of the unusual cross-sectional, axial views of the brain produced by CT requires considerable topographical anatomical reorientation. Unlike in conventional X-rays, the skull is no longer the anatomical reference point used for identification and localization of normal anatomical structures and pathological changes found in the intracranial space. In CT the brain itself with its relative densities, CSF spaces, gray and white matter, dural structures, and blood vessels provides structural points of topographical reference.

Over the years, a familiarization with the formerly unaccustomed CT imaging has taken place. Other more recent image processing techniques (90) for sectional visualization of biological structures will necessitate similar guidelines for the evaluation of pathological findings.

2.1 CT Technique

In CT, a slice of the examined body is visualized on a cathode ray tube (CRT) using X-ray transmission. Finely grouped X-ray beams scan the object to be examined in a circular fashion. Slight differences in the absorption coefficient or in intensities of the remnant radiation are measured by a detector system. The scan rotates around the subject either in "translation-rotation" steps or according to a quanta X-ray beam system. The absorption coefficients measured in a cross section of the body and their spatial arrangement are translated into gray scale values in a matrix format on a CRT (225). This can only be accomplished with an expensive measuring apparatus and a complicated computing procedure.

CT is a mathematical reconstruction rather than a direct image. It shows structures with different X-ray densities and contour deformations of organs or their inherent parts. Primary isodense pathological regions can be identified only through their altered perfusion following administration of a contrast medium (239). Although the density resolution of CT exceeds that of conventional X-ray techniques, the geometrical resolution remains inferior despite the greater number of detectors and higher resolution matrix.

The density measurements taken from a chosen region play a major role in the actual imaging processing. The absorption coefficients (remnant radiation) of a tissue section can be given in Hounsfield units (HU) and can be arranged according to specific standard values. The available gray scales of the monitor image do not permit satisfactory visual differentiation of the clinically interesting structures when the entire scale is used. For this reason, an electronic manipulation of the monitor image is necessary for observation and evaluation of the structures scanned. By selecting the "window width" and "window level or center", the available gray scales of the monitor image are adjusted to the radiodensity of special interest. A broad "window width" makes the bony structures appear extremely "plastic". A narrow window improves recognition of structures, such as the brain substance, with only slightly different densities.

The CT technique is limited by the measuring precision of the system, which may produce anatomical inaccuracies. Especially relevant to the reproductive accuracy of CT images is the partial volume effect. The gray values of the monitor image represent the average of all measured compartmental densities of one volume unit. A large difference in the densities of adjacent structures in one volume unit leads to a misinterpretation of these component densities, and hence to a misrepresentation of the structural borders, a masking of interstitial spaces as well as a coarser illustration and distortion of these structures. The partial volume effect can be reduced by using higher resolution matrices and examining thinner sections. This effect, along with artifacts and varying conditions of each examination, i.e., introduction of a contrast agent, positioning and movement of the examined object, influence the CT examination and must be considered in the evaluation of the resulting images (199, 313).

Over the past few years, faster computer analysis of

measured data has reduced the time of examination, and thereby made possible angiocomputed tomography. Intravenous injection or infusion of an iodine containing contrast agent enables imaging of small cranial vessels (116, 322, 323, 324).

2.2 Positron Emission Tomography

In positron emission tomography (PET) radioactive substances are usually injected intravenously into the patients to be examined. The positron emission tomography is a computed tomographic variation of classical scintigraphy (141). Two types of positron emission tomography exist. One type is a single-photon scanner (268), which utilizes a rotating gamma camera; the other uses a β^+ nuclide beam (330). In both instances, a three-dimensional sectional image technique shows the distribution of the injected radioactive tracer. In this way, metabolic processes, vascularization of organs and their subdivisions as well as tumors can be measured (19, 115, 123, 129, 291).

2.3 Ultrasound Techniques

Ultrasound techniques initially produced only a one-dimensional A-image (A-scan) for the identification of structure and organ boundaries. In recent years, ultrasound waves have been used in a process called sonography to produce sectional images that show morphological tissue characteristics. These sonographic images are known as B-scans. Because of the high absorption of sound waves by the skull and the difficult physical implementation of ultrasound technique, the brain cannot be visualized after closure of the fontanelles. In neurological examinations of newborns and small children sonography has become an increasingly important sectional image processing technique (22, 23, 68, 178, 227). Compound scanning apparatuses are available; these produce static images with a high resolution. Disadvantages of this technique in examinations of the brain include its relatively clumsy and inconvenient method of application and its limited mobility. Unlike the images produced by the real-time apparatus, static sonographic images do not show vascular pulsation. Real-time apparatuses are classified as either parallel or sector scan instruments. All these can be applied to infants in their first months and premature babies with their physiological acoustic window (anterior fontanelle) still open. The parallel scanner provides a good general outline of the ventricular system. The area of the brain demonstrated by this method is, however, limited by the width of the fontanelle or sagittal suture (288).

The sector scanner, however, can depict a large portion of the cranial cavity through a small, almost closed window, because of the wide-divergence quality of the ultrasound waves. Real-time apparatuses are easy to maneuver and the ultrasound waves are non-ionizing, making this technique suitable for the use on pediatric wards and premature infant units. In certain clinical settings this technique may supplement or even replace conventional X-ray studies and computed tomography (274, 292, 307). Advantages of the ultrasound technique are the clear depiction of borderline structures between different tissues and the choice of cross-sectional planes (73). Ultrasound procedures have been developed recently in a translation-rotation technique for the representation of soft tissues. Presently such techniques are not applicable to the brain (121, 275).

2.4 Magnetic Resonance Imaging
(Figs. 1b and c)

Over the past years, increasing clinical interest has been shown in magnetic resonance (MR) imaging (3, 20, 29, 182, 218, 252, 315). The introduction of this technique represents a new diagnostic tool that employs magnetic and high-frequency fields instead of ionizing radiation. An image is produced based on the magnetic effect of the spin (angular momentum) of atomic nuclei with an odd atomic number (number of protons plus neutrons). Hydrogen has an unusually large spin. In water, the most abundant biological substance, two hydrogen atoms are bound with one atom of oxygen. As a result, water is especially well shown in MR imaging. Lipids and proteins, however, are also easy to identify (83, 89, 92, 129, 326, 327). Each chemical element has a specific and unique resonance spin density spectrum. Another unique characteristic of each element is the relaxation time spectrum produced by the vibration decay times of the excited atoms as the nuclei return to their normal state. The signal used to produce the MR image is a function of proton density and relaxation time. The results obtained are influenced considerably by the measuring parameters chosen (60, 61). The processing of the measured data into gray scale values or color scales corresponds with that of conventional computed tomography. The resulting image depends on the chosen method of examination and the technical data of the apparatus used. Due to the absence of overlapping adjacent bony structures in MR images, lesions in the infratentorial compartment or of the basal portions of the cerebrum are often represented more clearly than in conventional computed tomography.

Initial clinical experience shows that foci typical of multiple sclerosis, which often escape identification

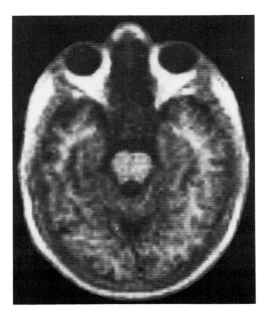

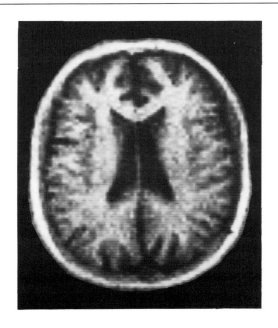

Figs. 1b, c Two MR images of the head of a 43-year-old male as seen approximately in the infraorbitomeatal sectioning plane. The reconstruction is achieved by the inversion-recovery mode.

Fig. 1b shows the eyeball and the retrobulbar fat in the orbit along with the basilar portions of the temporal lobes and the brain stem in the middle and posterior cranial fossa.

Fig. 1c illustrates the telencephalon at the level of the lateral ventricle with the central part. The frontal and occipital interhemispheric fissure can be identified.

with computed tomography, can be detected by MR (182, 326).

As in computed tomography, MR has a relatively poor geometrical resolution. In addition to axial and coronal sectional views, sagittal views of the brain can be obtained with MR without repositioning the patient. In the future, application of stronger magnetic fields and magnetic contrast materials with their distribution throughout the sectional images may provide information about such biochemical processes as tissue metabolism. For this purpose, MR-spectroscopy will be of particular importance and much is to be expected from phosphor-MR-spectroscopy (252).

2.5 CT Guideline Structures

A CT guideline structure is an easily detectable and generally reproducible part or compartment of the head, which serves as topical orientation for cranial computed tomography.

Each of the older neuroradiological techniques used in neurological diagnosis, pneumoencephalography and angiography show a specific anatomical system. Deformation of CSF spaces, as well as displacement and changes of cerebral blood vessels, may be signs of pathological processes. The general picture of the radiologically contrasted structures and their relative position to the skull serve as topical orientation.

Computed tomography reproduces images of the brain depicting different anatomical structures. Such an image is possible primarily due to its high density resolution. The amount of information obtained from this technique is greater than that provided by previous radiological techniques. However, the geometrical or spatial resolution of small structures is inferior to that of conventional X-ray images and, among other factors, depends considerably on the matrix chosen. The range of absorption coefficients, on which gray values are based, is related to measurements taken from biologically important structures of the head. Air, which appears black, has the lowest absorption coefficient at −1000 Hounsfield units (HU). Water has an absorption set at zero, while dense bone, which appears white, is set at approximately +1000 units (69, 235, 313). A head scan (170, 199, 313) will differentiate the following structures with the corresponding absorption coefficients:

Air	up to –1000 HU
Fatty tissue	–30 to –100 HU
CSF spaces	+5 to +10 HU
Gray and white cerebral matter	+20 to +40 HU
Blood vessels with contrast medium	+50 to +90 HU
Calcifications	+80 to +200 HU
Skull	+200 to +1000 HU and above

In the region of the facial bones and skull base, the bony structures and the air-filled paranasal sinuses serve as useful points of orientation. Intracranially, the CSF spaces and the varying densities of cerebral matter act as a frame of reference for the topographical arrangement of neuroanatomical structures. It should be pointed out, however, that in the vicinity of the skull base cerebral details may appear indistinct due to frequent artifacts. By choosing thinner sections for examination and specific sectioning planes, the formation of artifacts can be kept to a minimum. Dural structures, especially the cerebral falx and the tentorium of the cerebellum, are constantly visible guidelines. This is also true for the pineal gland and the choroid plexus of the lateral ventricles. These structures commonly calcify in early adulthood. Because of its almost identical absorption coefficient with the cerebral matter, the intracranial vascular system is not visualized in normal CT scans and is therefore of no importance as a guideline structure. In postinfusion CT scans, however, large vessels can be demonstrated. In angio-computed tomography (322, 323, 324), utilizing a quick scanner, a bolus injection of contrast medium, a high resolution technique, and an appropriate sectioning plane permit visualization of cerebral vessels.

2.5.1 Craniocervical Junction

(Figs. 19, 20, 5a, 6a)

The guideline structures in this region are the occipital bone with the foramen magnum and the upper portion of the vertebral column including the atlas and the dens of axis. Visible adjacent to the bony structures are the medulla oblongata and surrounding subarachnoid space, including the large and highly variable cisterna magna (cerebellomedullary cistern). The cerebellar tonsils and the medulla oblongata form a characteristic Y-shaped figure. In a postinfusion scan, the vertebral arteries and the

epidural venous plexus are seen. Through intrathecal application of contrast media deformations of the subarachnoid space can be shown clearly.

2.5.2 Base of the Skull

(Figs. 20–23 and 6a–9a)

Structural points of orientation are the bones of the skull base, the intermediary spaces, and the cisterns. They all supply information concerning the choice and position of the sectioning plane used in the examination. Crude orientation is provided by the occipital bones, petrous bones, mastoid (air) cells, sphenoid sinus, sella turcica, ethmoidal cells (sinus), zygomatic arches, and orbital borders. Other structures, which are not constantly shown in CT images of the skull base, are the hypoglossal canal, jugular foramen, internal acoustic (auditory) meatus, tympanic cavity, foramen lacerum, carotid canal, spinous foramen, and oval foramen. Detailed perspectives of the base are obtained by examining thinner sections, deviating from the canthomeatal plane, and by imaging the brain with additional coronal scans. Due to higher geometrical resolution, conventional X-rays of the bony structures of the craniocervical junction and the skull base, made from anatomical sections, provide more detailed images than those of X-ray computed tomography. For this reason, we chose X-rays for the depiction of the anatomy of the skull base (Figs. 20–23).

2.5.3 Visceral Cranium

The facial bones serve as important points of reference for the interpretation of cranial CT images. The paranasal sinuses, ramus of the mandible, zygomatic bones, and mastoid (air) cells are constant guideline structures. Teeth, especially those with metal fillings, can produce disturbing artifacts. In higher sections, ethmoidal cells, the bones forming the orbit, and the soft tissues of the orbit are regularly identifiable. The sectioning plane in the orbital region usually lies at a 10° angle to the canthomeatal plane (119), thereby approximating the infraorbitomeatal plane (Chap. 1.4). In this way the optic nerve and extraocular muscles are better shown. By letting the patient look slightly upward, the normally coiled optic nerve is straightened (199, 313). Lens, sclera, and vitreous body of the ocular bulb are consistently visible. The lacrimal gland is often hidden by the upper lid.

2.5.4 Cisterns and Ventricular System (Figs. 25, 26, 27)

In the intracranial compartment, the CSF spaces are the important points of reference. Only the enlarged areas of the subarachnoid space are depicted in CT scans (170). Fine fissural spaces are hidden by other denser structures or are simply averaged out by the partial volume effect. Identifiable, however, are the unpaired cisterna magna (cerebellomedullary cistern) and pontine cistern and the paired cerebellopontine (angle) cisterns. These spaces are located at the level of the petrous portion of the temporal bone in a plane approximately parallel to the supraorbitomeatal plane (Chap. 1.4). Immediately above these guideline structures are the anterior basal cistern, interpeduncular cistern, and superior cerebellar cistern. According to Hilal (120), the suprasellar cistern or "pentagon", a pentahedral structure in CT images, is formed by the medial frontal basal cistern and the interpeduncular cistern. It encircles the infundibulum, optic nerves, and optic chiasm.

The frontal boundary of the suprasellar cistern is the gyrus rectus. It borders laterally on the uncus and parahippocampal gyrus and occipitally on the pons. Additional important CSF spaces of reference are the ambient cistern and cistern of tectal lamina. In young patients, the insular cisterns and those located in the interhemispheric fissure are very narrow. These CSF spaces, however, are especially well seen in older patients and in those suffering from cerebral atrophy. Detailed images of the cisterns are obtained by introducing a suitable water-soluble contrast agent, such as Metrizamide, through lumbar puncture into the subarachnoid space.

Due to the great physiological variability of the width of the ventricular system and its flexible adaptation in the presence of displacing tumors, no consistent reproductions of the individual subdivisions of the ventricles are available. The temporal horns are frequently undetectable. Images with wide bilateral temporal horns, indicate hydrocephalus (293). The volume of the ventricular system is calculated according to surface area measurements of the ventricles taken from several CT images (30, 93, 191, 242, 255, 328).

2.5.5 Blood Vessels (Figs. 5a–18a)

Without a contrast medium, the cranial blood vessels are not constantly identifiable. Segments of the basilar and internal carotid arteries can occasionally be identified in normal CT scans. With a special technique, more vessels can be seen, such as those in the orbit (314). In postinfusion CT scans, the middle cerebral artery and its branches in the lateral sulcus, portions of the internal carotid arteries, segments of the circle of Willis, and the basilar artery can generally be demonstrated. Venous guideline structures are the great cerebral vein (Galen), inferior sagittal sinus, straight sinus, and superior sagittal sinus. The transverse sinus, on the other hand, is seen only occasionally (202).

2.5.6 Dura Mater (Figs. 5b–18b)

The dura mater (pachymeninx) cannot or only rarely be detected in CT scans. Dura duplications are usually clearly evident. The cerebral falx is constantly shown in postinfusion CT scans, because the superior and inferior sagittal sinuses along with the straight sinus and smaller bridging veins are visualized in the venous phase, thereby forming a border around the entire cerebral falx. The tentorium of cerebellum is usually distinctly demarcated only after infusion of a contrast agent (214). It is bounded below and laterally by the confluence of sinuses, namely the transverse sinus, parts of the straight sinus, the superior petrosal sinus and its free edge running toward the anterior clinoid process. The topographical location of the tentorial notch (incisura) to the midbrain varies widely. Images of sections through the tentorium and cerebral falx can take on a Y-shape (Figs. 11b.40 and 12b.40). Sectional images of the tentorium appear V- or M-shaped. The tentorial notch (incisura) is indicated in postinfusion CT scans by the ventromedial segments of the diverging bands (201).

When the tentorium cannot be visualized in normal axial CT scans, the diverging bands can be constructed using an auxiliary line. This line extends from the lateral portion of the ambient cistern (not from the medial part of the cistern of the tectal lamina) in an occipital-lateral direction toward the skull and lies at a 45° angle to the sagittal plane. Structures lateral to this auxiliary line are located supratentorial. Those on the medial side lie infratentorial (201). In coronal sections, the tentorium of cerebellum is usually clearly visible.

2.5.7 Brain Structures
(Figs. 6b–18b)

The differentiation of gray and white matter of the brain is made possible by the excellent high density resolution of computed tomography. Therefore, the demarcation of the putamen, caudate nucleus, globus pallidus, and other nuclei can be accomplished. These CT guideline structures, furthermore, render possible a spatial localization of smaller anatomical structures, neurofunctional systems, and pathological intracranial structures.

3 Topography of the Cranial Cavity, Cerebrospinal Fluid Spaces, Arteries, Veins, Cranial Nerves, and Subdivisions of the Brain as Seen in the Canthomeatal Parallel Planes

Topography describes the position of anatomical structures in space. Standard textbooks of cranial topography (Chap. 1.5), written before the development of computed tomography, depicted anatomical structures as conceived from the individual layers of a sectioned brain. Much of the information was gained from neurosurgery.

In neuroanatomy, the use of computed tomography requires a special three-dimensional knowledge of anatomical structures in order to interpret parallel brain slices. Similar to the architect's conception of an entire building and its subunits using the plans of sequential floors, the equidistant serial CT cross sections of the head provide the neurologist with an illustration of the anatomical structures. Unlike the precise architectural drawings, in which right angles predominate, however, CT scans produce highly variable contours due to the complex shapes of anatomical structures.

The position of the individual slices in serial sections is especially important for the identification of the anatomical structures included. Figure 2 is a lateral view of the head showing the X-ray dense structures and the positions of the 14 slices. The positions of the 14 slices of the spinal cord and the brain are shown in a medial (Fig. 3) and a lateral view (Fig. 4). Figures 5 to 18 are illustrations of the individual slices. Each slice with its structures is numbered and viewed from the top in Figures 5 to 18. The depicted surface of each section (Figs. 5 to 18) represents the line above the encircled number of the corresponding slice in Figures 1a, 2, 3, 4. The advantages and disadvantages of the various cross-sectional parallel planes used in CT examinations of the human brain are discussed in Chapter 1.4.

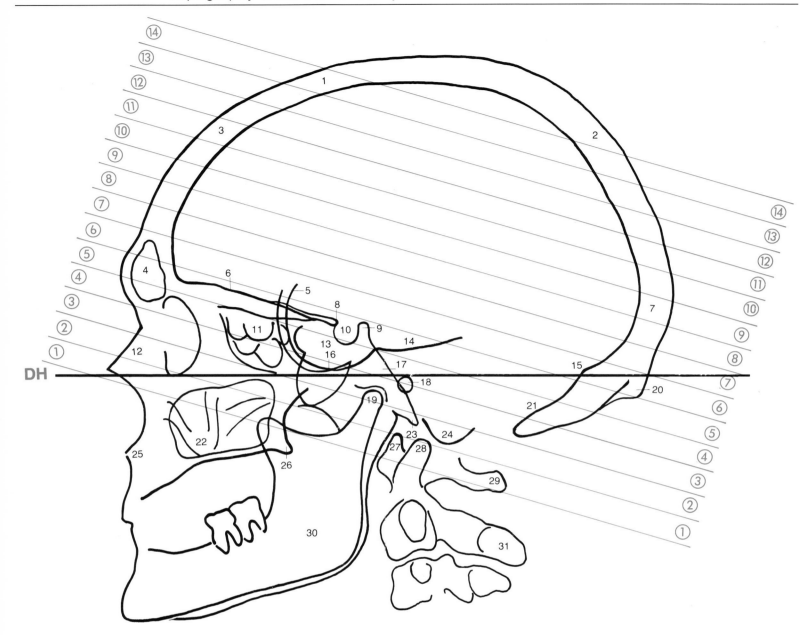

Fig. 2 Lateral X-ray of the head of a 44-year-old male (see Chap. 1.3). The 14 slices were assembled in their original anatomical locations and numbered continuously in a caudal to cranial direction. The encircled number indicates the number of the slice.
DH = Reid's base line = "Deutsche Horizontale".

1 Bregma
2 Parietal bone
3 Frontal bone
4 Frontal sinus
5 Greater wing of sphenoid bone
6 Floor of anterior cranial fossa
7 Occipital bone
8 Anterior clinoid process
9 Dorsum sellae, posterior clinoid process
10 Sella turcica (pituitary fossa)

11 Ethmoidal cells (sinus)
12 Nasal bone
13 Sphenoid sinus
14 Superior margin of petrous bone
15 Internal occipital protuberance
16 Floor of middle cranial fossa
17 Clivus
18 External acoustic (auditory) meatus
19 Head of mandible
20 External occipital protuberance (inion)

21 Floor of posterior cranial fossa
22 Maxillary sinus
23 Basion
24 Mastoid process
25 Anterior nasal spine
26 Posterior nasal spine
27 Anterior arch of atlas
28 Dens of axis
29 Posterior arch of atlas
30 Mandible
31 Spinous process of axis

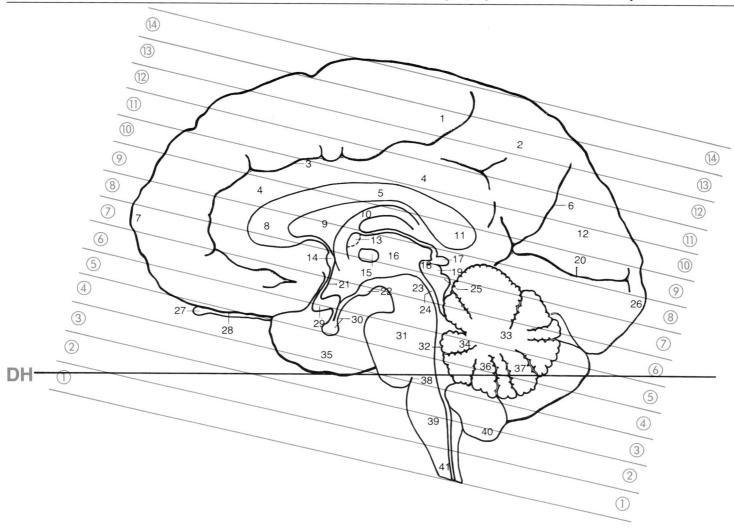

Fig. 3 Medial view of the brain of a 44-year-old male (see Chap. 1.3). The slices were fitted back together and numbered as shown in Figure 2.
DH = Reid's base line = "Deutsche Horizontale".

1 Paracentral lobule
2 Precuneus
3 Cingulate sulcus
4 Cingulate gyrus
5 Trunk of corpus callosum
6 Parieto-occipital sulcus
7 Frontal pole
8 Genu of corpus callosum
9 Septum pellucidum
10 Fornix
11 Splenium of corpus callosum
12 Cuneus
13 Interventricular foramen (Monro)
14 Anterior commissure

15 Interthalamic adhesion (intermediate mass)
16 Third ventricle
17 Pineal gland (pineal body, epiphysis)
18 Posterior commissure
19 Superior colliculus
20 Calcarine sulcus
21 Lamina terminalis
22 Mamillary body
23 Mesencephalon
24 Aqueduct
25 Inferior colliculus
26 Occipital pole
27 Olfactory bulb

28 Olfactory tract
29 Optic chiasm
30 Infundibulum and hypophysis
31 Pons
32 Fourth ventricle
33 Cerebellum
34 Nodule of vermis
35 Temporal lobe
36 Uvula of vermis
37 Pyramis of vermis
38 Foramen cecum
39 Medulla oblongata
40 Tonsil of cerebellum
41 Spinal cord

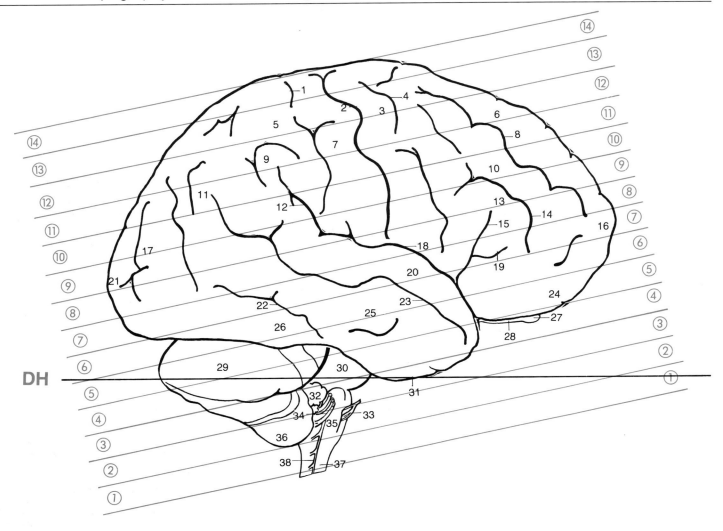

Fig. 4 Lateral view of the brain of a 44-year-old male (see Chap. 1.3.). The slices were fitted back together and numbered as shown in Figure 2.
DH = Reid's base line = "Deutsche Horizontale".

1 Postcentral sulcus
2 Central sulcus
3 Precentral gyrus
4 Precentral sulcus
5 Superior parietal lobule
6 Superior frontal gyrus
7 Postcentral gyrus
8 Superior frontal sulcus
9 Supramarginal gyrus
10 Middle frontal gyrus
11 Angular gyrus
12 Posterior branch of lateral sulcus
13 Inferior frontal gyrus
14 Inferior frontal sulcus

15 Ascending branch of lateral sulcus
16 Frontal pole
17 Occipital gyri
18 Lateral sulcus (Sylvian fissure)
19 Anterior branch of lateral sulcus
20 Superior temporal gyrus
21 Occipital pole
22 Inferior temporal sulcus
23 Superior temporal sulcus
24 Orbital gyri
25 Middle temporal gyrus
26 Inferior temporal gyrus

27 Olfactory bulb
28 Olfactory tract
29 Cerebellum
30 Pons
31 Base of temporal lobe
32 Flocculus
33 Hypoglossal nerve
34 Glossopharyngeal nerve, vagus nerve, and accessory nerve
35 Medulla oblongata
36 Tonsil of cerebellum
37 Spinal cord
38 Spinal root of accessory nerve

3.1 Cranial Cavity (Figs. 5–18 and 25)

Located inside a rigid capsule, the cranial cavity is a hollow space with an average volume of 1550 ml in males and 1425 ml in females (56). Inside this cavity, the brain with its nerves and vessels floats in a liquid medium, the cerebrospinal fluid (CSF). Rigid sheets of dura mater divide the cranial cavity into separate compartments. The tentorium of cerebellum (Figs. 9b.19, 10b.40, 11b.40, 12b.40) divides the cranial cavity into a supratentorial and an infratentorial compartment. The floor of the infratentorial compartment is the posterior cranial fossa, and its roof is shaped like a shallow-pitched tent by the tentorium of cerebellum. The brain stem emerges through a large oval-shaped opening called the tentorial notch (incisura). A fluid jacket, the ambient cistern, is found here (Chap. 3.2). The foramen magnum is the other large opening of the infratentorial compartment (Fig. 6a.20). It can be oval or almost circular in shape, usually giving the appearance of two differently sized semicircles placed together. The area of the foramen magnum averages 8 cm^2, ranging from 5–10 cm^2. In cases of extreme cerebral edema, the brain stem and the cerebellum are pushed into a more caudal position. As a result, a pressure cone may develop on the caudal surface of the cerebellum and may cause tonsillar herniation.

The supratentorial compartment is partially divided by the sickle-shaped cerebral falx (Figs. 9b.1, 10b.3, 11b.3, 12b.3, 13b.3, 14b.3). Fluid jackets protect the neighboring structures of the cerebrum, namely the interhemispheric cistern and the pericallosal cistern. The subdivision of the cranial cavity into separate compartments by the fibrous sheets of dura mater determines the possibility and direction of a major displacement of the individual brain structures in the event of an increase in intracranial pressure. An increase in volume of the cerebrum in the supratentorial compartment may strangulate the brain stem giving rise to a midbrain syndrome.

Furthermore, a displacement in one hemisphere may bend the cerebral falx towards the opposite side. Knowledge of changes such as these is essential for both diagnosis and surgical intervention. When planning a neurosurgical procedure, the position of the blood vessels in the tentorium and cerebral falx must be taken into consideration in order to avoid unnecessary hemorrhagic complications (Chaps. 3.3 and 3.4).

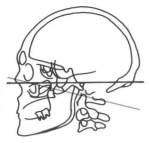

1 Nasal bone
2 Nasal septum
3 Maxilla
4 Orbit
5 Zygomatic bone
6 Infraorbital canal
7 Maxillary sinus
8 Palatine bone
9 Lateral lamina of pterygoid
    process
10 Mandible
11 Internal carotid artery
12 Styloid process
13 Internal jugular vein
14 Anterior arch of atlas
15 Dens of axis
16 Occipital condyle
17 Lateral mass of atlas
18 Auricle (pinna)
19 Vertebral artery,
    V3 segment
20 Posterior arch of atlas

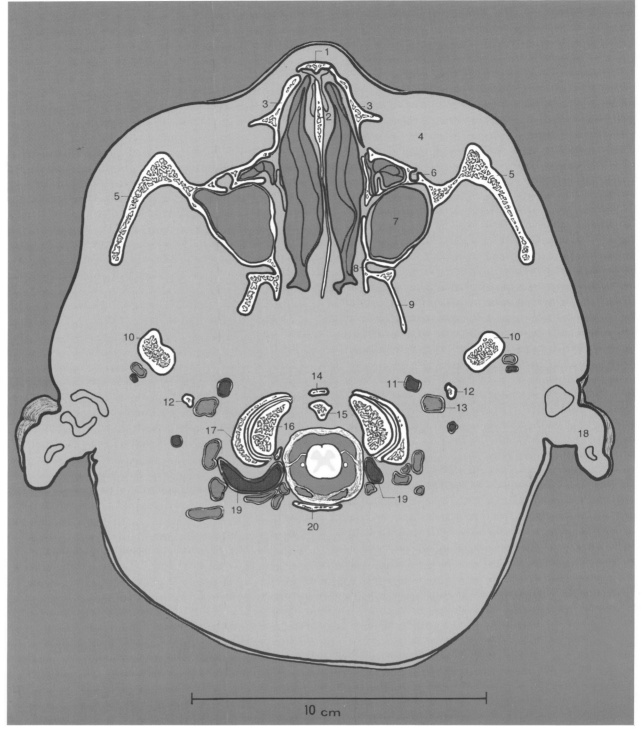

Fig. 5a Cranial sectioning surface of the first slice. In the upper left hand corner of the page, the blue line through the lateral X-ray view of the skull indicates the position of the sectioning plane through the craniocervical junction at the level of the occipital ccndyles and the atlas (compare with Fig. 2). Bony structures and blood vessels.

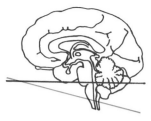

1 Anterior median fissure
2 Ventral root of the first spinal nerve
3 Spinal cord
4 Spinal root of accessory nerve
5 Dorsal funiculus
6 Dura mater

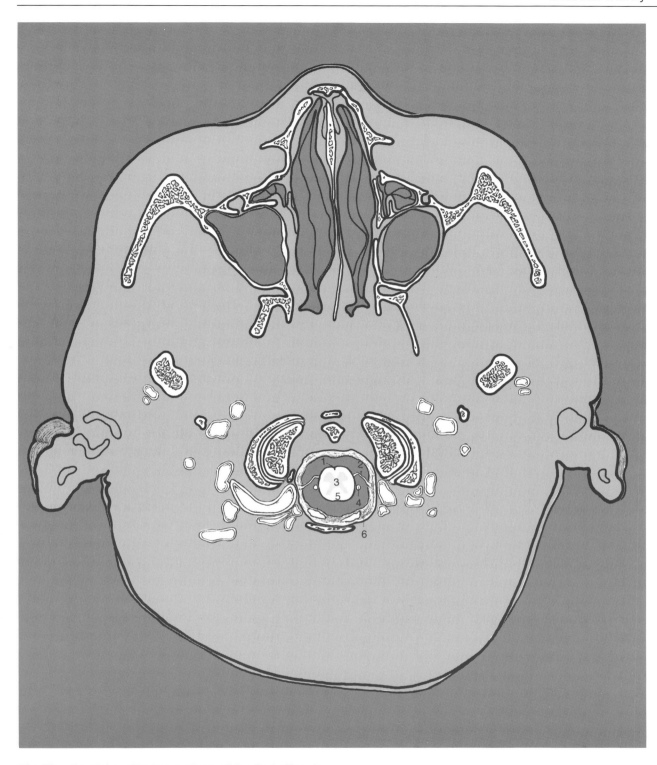

Fig. 5b Cranial sectioning surface of the first slice. In the upper right hand corner of the page, the blue line through the median view of the brain indicates the location of the sectioning plane through the spinal cord (see Fig. 3). Spinal cord and meninges.

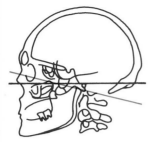

1 Nasal bone
2 Nasal septum
3 Zygomatic bone
4 Ethmoidal cells (sinus)
5 Orbit
6 Maxillary sinus
7 Zygomatic arch
8 Sphenoid sinus
9 Cartilage of auditory tube
10 Mandible
11 Basilar part of occipital
   bone
12 Internal carotid artery
13 Internal jugular vein
14 Floor of external acoustic
   meatus
15 Vertebral artery
16 Hypoglossal canal
17 Mastoid process
18 Posterior inferior cerebellar artery (PICA)
19 Auricle (pinna)
20 Foramen magnum

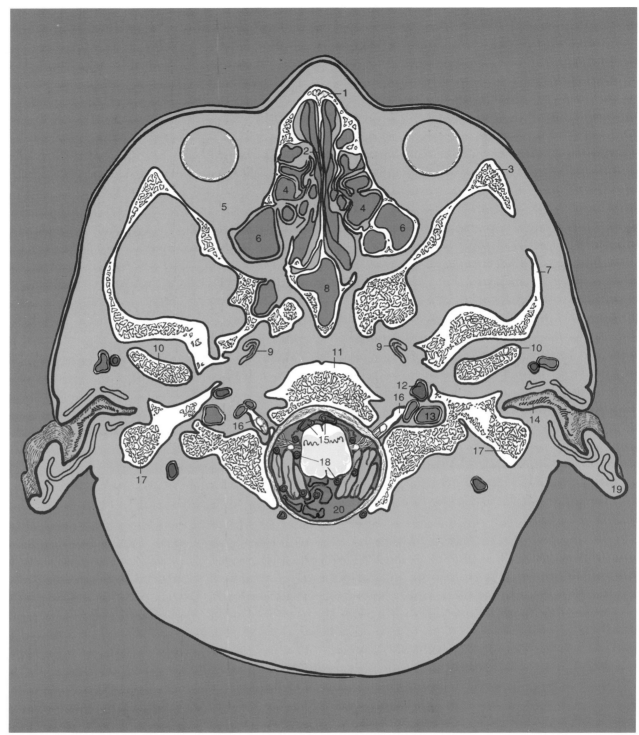

Fig. 6a Cranial sectioning surface of the second slice. The sectioning plane runs diagonally to the foramen magnum (see text) at the level of the hypoglossal canal. The floor of the lateral portion of the external acoustic (auditory) meatus is cut horizontally. Bony structures and blood vessels.

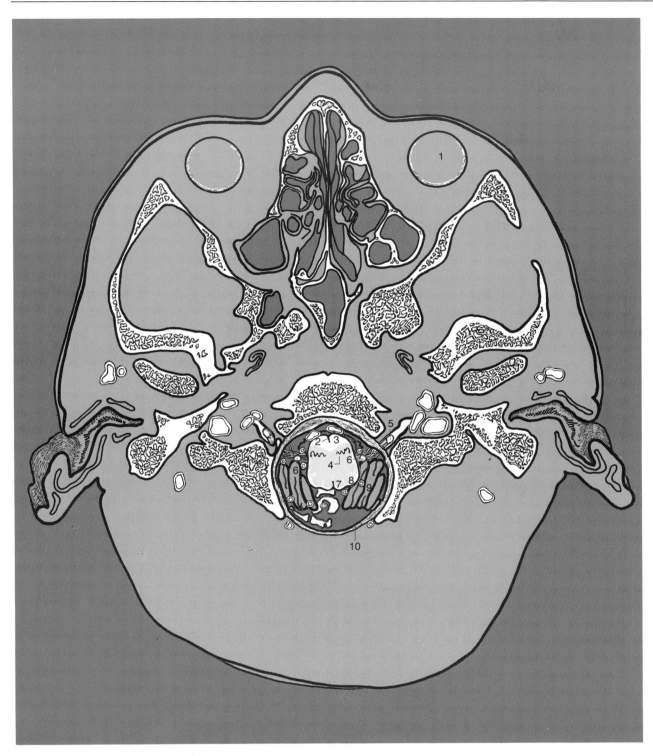

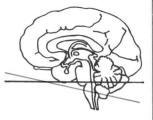

1 Ocular bulb
2 Anterior median fissure
3 Pyramid
4 Inferior olivary nucleus
5 Hypoglossal nerve
6 Spinal root of accessory nerve
7 Tubercle of gracile nucleus (Goll)
8 Tubercle of cuneate nucleus (Burdach)
9 Tonsil of cerebellum
10 Dura mater

Fig. 6b Cranial sectioning surface of the second slice. The posterior cranial fossa is cut just above the foramen magnum. The medulla oblongata and cerebellar tonsils are dissected. Brain structures and meninges.

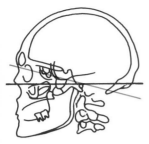

1 Ethmoidal cells (sinus)
2 Zygomatic bone
3 Ethmoid bone
4 Orbit
5 Sphenoid bone
6 Frontal branch of middle
  meningeal artery
7 Sphenoid sinus
8 Temporal bone
9 Internal carotid artery
10 Clivus
11 Basilar artery
12 Tympanic cavity
13 Tympanic membrane
14 External acoustic
   (auditory) meatus
15 Anterior inferior cerebellar
   artery (AICA)
16 Jugular foramen
17 Internal jugular vein
18 Facial canal
19 Sigmoid sinus
20 Mastoid (air) cells
21 Auricle (pinna)
22 Occipital sinus
23 Occipital bone

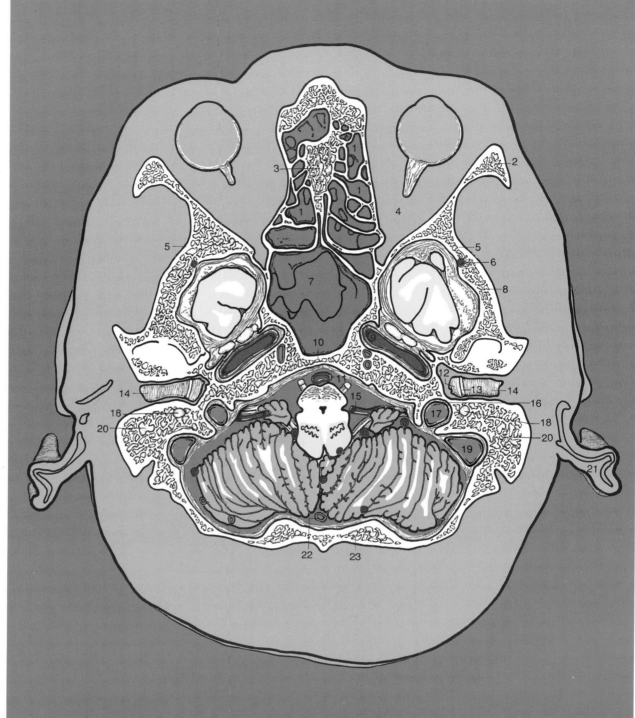

Fig. 7a Cranial sectioning surface of the third slice. The sectioning plane runs through the middle of the ocular bulbs and medial portion of the external acoustic (auditory) meatus. This corresponds to the cantho-meatal plane. The floor of the middle cranial fossa lies in the section just below the sectioning plane. X-ray of this section shows the oval foramen and the spinous foramen (Fig. 21). Bony structures and blood vessels.

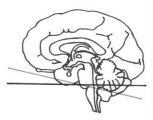

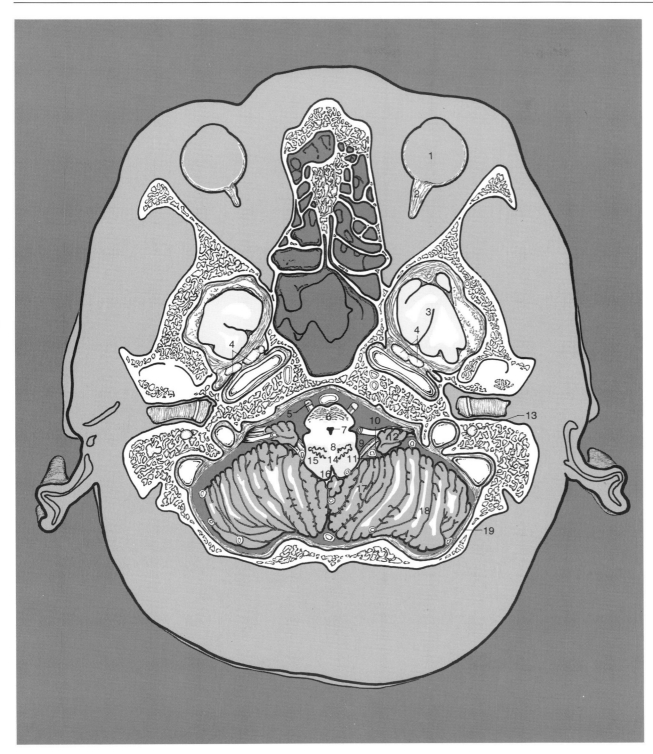

1 Ocular bulb
2 Optic nerve
3 Base of temporal lobe
4 Maxillary and mandibular
   nerves
5 Abducens nerve
6 Pons
7 Foramen cecum
8 Inferior olivary nucleus
9 Glossopharyngeal nerve
   and vagus nerve
10 Accessory nerve
11 Spinal root of accessory
   nerve
12 Flocculus
13 Facial nerve
14 Medulla oblongata
15 Tubercle of cuneate
   nucleus (Burdach)
16 Tubercle of gracile nucleus
   (Goll)
17 Tonsil of cerebellum
18 Hemisphere of posterior
   lobe
19 Dura mater

Fig. 7b Cranial sectioning surface of the third slice. The sectioning plane intersects the middle of the ocular bulbs and the base of both temporal lobes and cuts diagonally through the border between pons and medulla oblongata. The facial nerve is cut in the bony canal of the petrous bone. Brain structures and meninges.

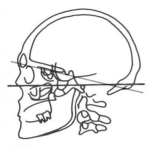

1 Frontal bone
2 Frontal sinus
3 Crista galli
4 Orbit
5 Sphenoid bone
6 Superior orbital fissure
7 Frontal branch of middle
  meningeal artery
8 Sphenoid sinus
9 Cavernous sinus
10 Internal carotid artery
11 Dorsum sellae (cut)
12 Basilar artery
13 Malleus (hammer)
14 Incus (anvil)
15 Internal acoustic (auditory)
   meatus
16 Tympanic cavity
17 Anterior semicircular canal
18 Anterior inferior cerebellar
   artery (AICA)
19 Temporal bone
20 Sigmoid sinus
21 Auricle (pinna)
22 Lambdoidal suture
23 Occipital sinus
24 Occipital bone

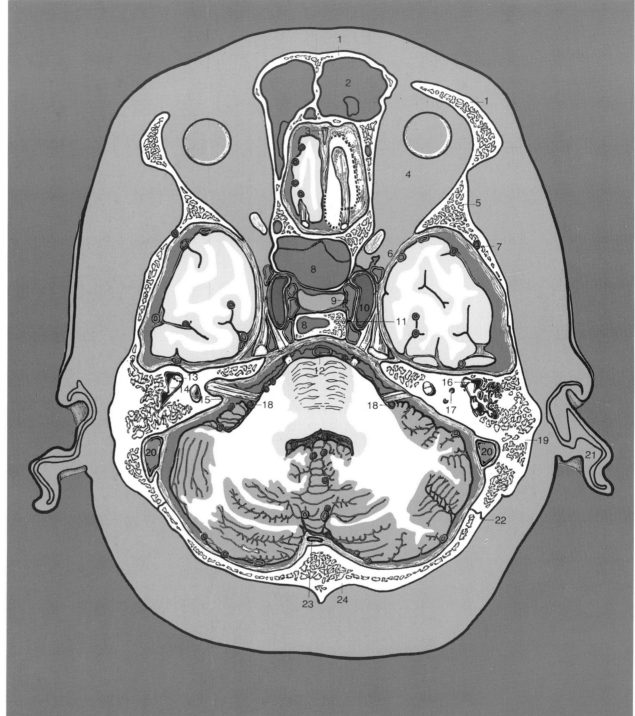

Fig. 8a Cranial sectioning surface cf the fourth slice. The recess in the anterior cranial fossa in the region of the cribriform plate is cut with basilar portions of the telencephalon. The sectioning plane cuts through the sella turcica and dissects the dorsum sellae. The posterior cranial fossa is shown with the internal acoustic (auditory) meatus. Bony structures and blood vessels.

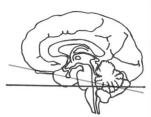

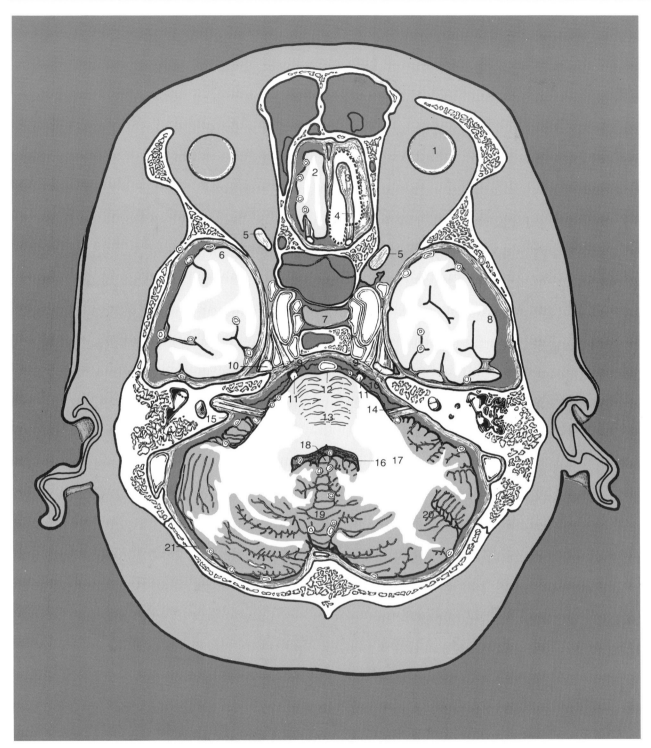

1 Ocular bulb
2 Gyrus rectus
3 Olfactory bulb
4 Olfactory tract
5 Optic nerve
6 Temporal lobe
7 Hypophysis (pituitary gland)
8 Inferior temporal gyrus
9 Abducens nerve
10 Trigeminal nerve
11 Abducens nerve near opening of dura mater
12 Basilar sulcus
13 Pons
14 Facial nerve and intermediate nerve (Wrisberg)
15 Vestibulocochlear nerve
16 Fourth ventricle
17 Middle cerebellar peduncle
18 Uvula of vermis
19 Vermis of cerebellum
20 Hemisphere of posterior lobe
21 Dura mater

Fig. 8b Cranial sectioning surface of the fourth slice. The frontal cortex covering the right half of the anterior cranial fossa has been removed to demonstrate the olfactory bulb and tract. These parts of the olfactory system are illustrated in the olfactory groove. The temporal lobes are shown in the middle cranial fossa. The pons and cerebellum are seen in the posterior cranial fossa. Brain structures and meninges.

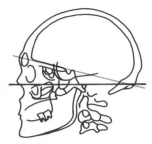

1 Frontal bone
2 Frontal sinus
3 Opened orbit
4 Anterior cranial fossa
5 Medial frontobasal artery
6 Sphenoid bone
7 Frontal branch of middle
  meningeal artery
8 Temporal artery
9 Anterior communicating
  artery
10 Anterior cerebral artery
11 Middle cerebral artery
12 Posterior communicating
  artery
13 Posterior cerebral artery
14 Basilar artery
15 Basal vein (Rosenthal)
16 Superior cerebellar artery
17 Tentorium of cerebellum
18 Temporal bone
19 Superior petrosal sinus
20 Sigmoid sinus
21 Auricle (pinna)
22 Lambdoidal suture
23 Occipital sinus
24 Internal occipital
  protuberance
25 Occipital bone
26 External occipital
  protuberance (inion)

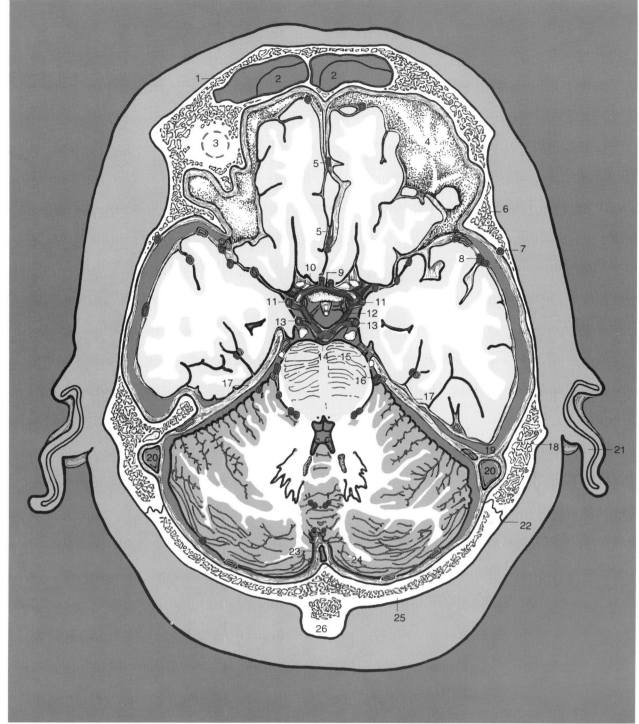

Fig. 9a Cranial sectioning surface of the fifth slice. The cerebral arterial circle (circle of Willis) was dissected and graphically reconstructed. On the left side the sectioning plane runs through the roof of the orbit and just above the dorsum sellae. The insertion of the tentorium of cerebellum covers both sides of the ventral portion of the superior margins of the petrous bones. Bony structures and blood vessels.

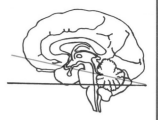

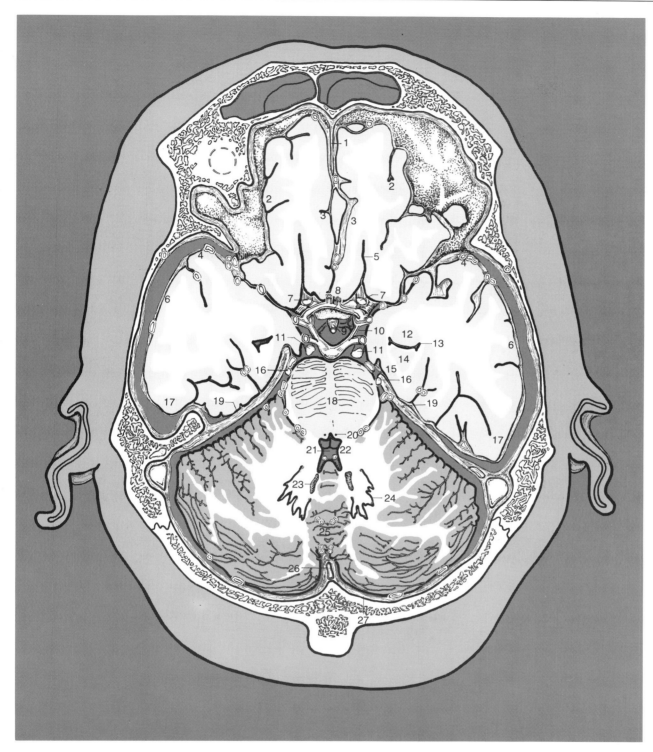

1 Cerebral falx
2 Orbital gyri
3 Gyrus rectus
4 Superior temporal gyrus
5 Olfactory sulcus
6 Middle temporal gyrus
7 Olfactory tract
8 Optic chiasm
9 Infundibulum
10 Posterior clinoid process
   (covered)
11 Oculomotor nerve
12 Amygdaloid body
   (nucleus)
13 Temporal horn of lateral
   ventricle
14 Hippocampal formation
15 Parahippocampal gyrus
16 Trochlear nerve
17 Inferior temporal gyrus
18 Pons
19 Tentorium of cerebellum
20 Locus ceruleus
21 Fourth ventricle
22 Superior cerebellar
   peduncle
23 Fastigial nucleus
24 Dentate nucleus
25 Vermis of cerebellum
26 Cerebellar falx
27 Dura mater

Fig. 9b   Cranial sectioning surface of the fifth slice.
The sectioning plane lies at the level of the entrance to
the sella. The frontal and temporal lobes, infundibulum,
pons, and cerebellum are shown. Brain structures and
meninges.

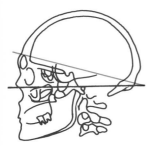

1 Frontal bone
2 Frontal sinus
3 Frontopolar artery
4 Branch of middle
   meningeal artery
5 Superficial middle cerebral
   vein
6 Anterior cerebral artery
7 Insular arteries
8 Temporal artery
9 Anterolateral central
   (lateral lenticulostriate (16))
   arteries
10 Anteromedial and
   anterolateral central
   (medial and lateral
   lenticulostriate (15, 16))
   arteries
11 Temporal bone
12 Medial occipital artery
13 Lateral occipital artery
14 Medial and lateral posterior
   choroid arteries
15 Basal vein (Rosenthal)
16 Auricle (pinna)
17 Tentorium of cerebellum
18 Lambdoidal suture
19 Transverse sinus
20 Occipital bone

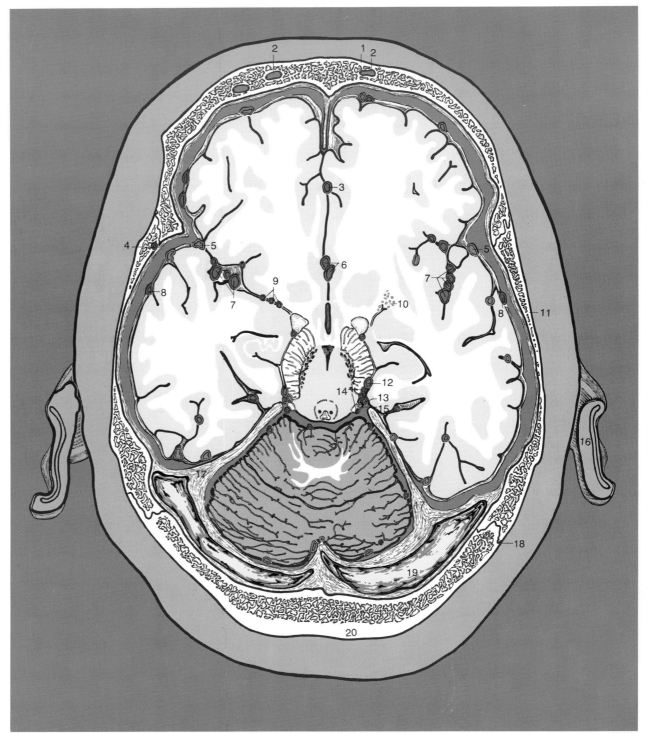

Fig. 10a   Cranial sectioning surface of the sixth slice showing the anterior, middle, and posterior cranial fossae with their structures. The tentorium of cerebellum forms the ventral border of the posterior cranial fossa. Bony structures and blood vessels.

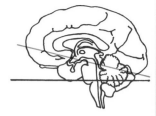

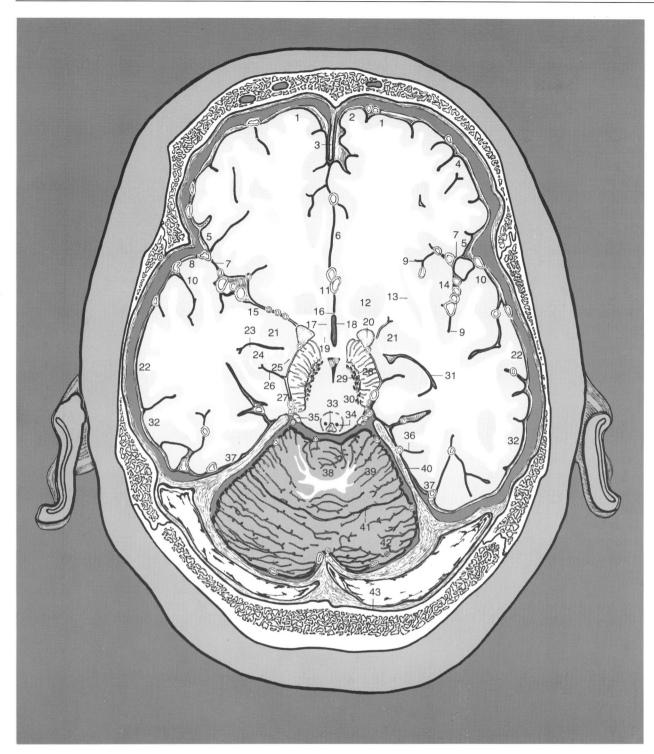

1 Superior frontal gyrus
2 Frontal pole
3 Cerebral falx
4 Middle frontal gyrus
5 Inferior frontal gyrus
6 Cingulate gyrus
7 Lateral sulcus (Sylvian fissure)
8 Temporal lobe
9 Circular sulcus of insula
10 Superior temporal gyrus
11 Subcallosal area
12 Floor of striatum
13 Claustrum
14 Insula (island of Reil)
15 Gyrus semilunaris
16 Lamina terminalis
17 Hypothalamus
18 Third ventricle
19 Fornix
20 Optic tract
21 Amygdaloid body (nucleus)
22 Middle temporal gyrus
23 Alveus
24 Hippocampus
25 Uncus of parahippocampal gyrus
26 Hippocampal sulcus
27 Parahippocampal gyrus
28 Base (ventral part) of cerebral peduncle
29 Substantia nigra
30 Tegmentum of mesencephalon
31 Temporal horn of lateral ventricle
32 Inferior temporal gyrus
33 Transition of aqueduct into the fourth ventricle
34 Locus ceruleus
35 Trochlear nerve
36 Collateral sulcus
37 Lateral occipitotemporal gyrus
38 Vermis of anterior lobe of cerebellum
39 Hemisphere of anterior lobe
40 Tentorium of cerebellum
41 Primary fissure
42 Hemisphere of posterior lobe
43 Dura mater

Fig. 10b Cranial sectioning surface of the sixth slice showing the frontal and temporal lobes, hypothalamus, mesencephalon, and cerebellum. Brain structures and meninges.

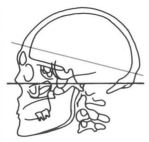

1 Frontal bone
2 Superior sagittal sinus
3 Bridging vein
4 Anteromedial (anterior internal (128)) frontal artery
5 Anterior cerebral artery
6 Insular arteries
7 Coronal suture
8 Parietal bone
9 Superficial middle cerebral vein
10 Temporal artery
11 Frontal horn of lateral ventricle
12 Anterolateral central (lateral lenticulostriate (16)) arteries
13 Third ventricle
14 Temporal bone
15 Medial occipital artery
16 Medial and lateral posterior choroid arteries
17 Aqueduct
18 Lateral occipital artery
19 Basal vein (Rosenthal)
20 Auricle (pinna)
21 Tentorium of cerebellum
22 Branch of lateral occipital artery
23 Straight sinus
24 Lambdoidal suture
25 Confluence of sinuses (blue dotted line within the slice)
26 Occipital bone

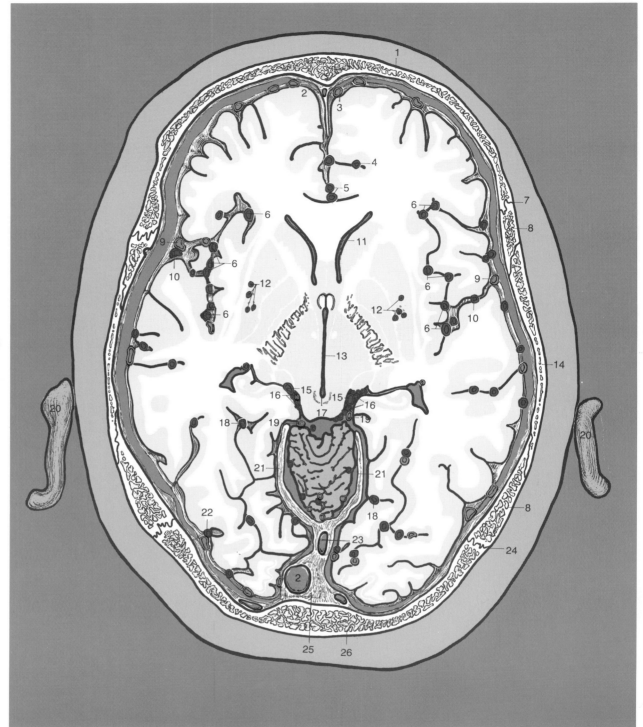

Fig. 11a Cranial sectioning surface of the seventh slice showing the basal portions of the frontal horns of the lateral ventricles. The third ventricle is cut as it merges into the aqueduct. The temporal horns of the lateral ventricles are also depicted. The ventral portion of the tentorium of cerebellum is dissected. Bony structures and blood vessels.

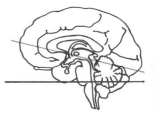

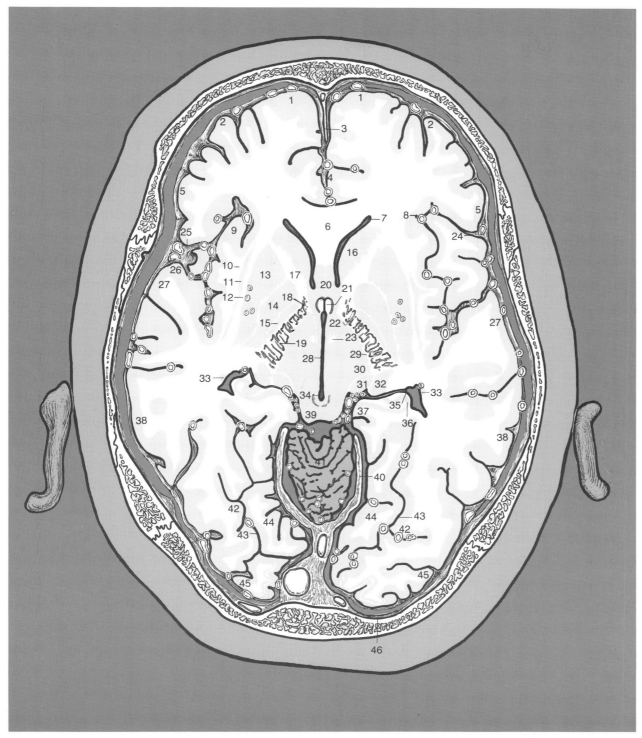

1 Superior frontal gyrus at the frontal pole
2 Middle frontal gyrus
3 Cerebral falx
✓4 Cingulate gyrus
5 Inferior frontal gyrus
6 Genu of corpus callosum
7 Frontal horn of lateral ventricle
8 Circular sulcus of insula
9 Insula (island of Reil)
10 Extreme capsule
11 Claustrum
12 External capsule
13 Putamen
14 Lateral part of globus pallidus
15 Medial part of globus pallidus
16 Head of caudate nucleus
17 Anterior limb (crus) of internal capsule
18 Genu of internal capsule
19 Posterior limb (crus) of internal capsule
20 Septum verum
✓21 Column of fornix
✓22 Hypothalamus
23 Mamillothalamic tract (Vicq d'Azyr)
24 Ascending branch of lateral sulcus
25 Posterior branch of lateral sulcus
26 Temporal lobe
✓27 Superior temporal gyrus
28 Third ventricle
29 Reticular nucleus of thalamus
30 Ventral posterolateral nucleus of thalamus (nucleus ventrocaudalis externus (107))
31 Medial geniculate body
32 Lateral geniculate body
33 Tail of caudate nucleus
34 Aqueduct
35 Alveus
36 Hippocampus
37 Parahippocampal gyrus
✓38 Middle temporal gyrus
39 Inferior colliculus
40 Tentorium of cerebellum
41 Vermis of anterior lobe of cerebellum
42 Lateral occipitotemporal gyrus
43 Collateral sulcus
44 Medial occipitotemporal gyrus
45 Occipital gyri
46 Dura mater

Fig. 11b Cranial sectioning surface of the seventh slice. In this plane, the insula reaches its greatest expansion. The striatum (putamen and caudate nucleus), internal capsule, hypothalamus, and caudal thalamus are depicted. In the infratentorial space, the cerebellum is shown only. Brain structures and meninges.

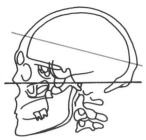

1 Frontal bone
2 Superior sagittal sinus
3 Superior (superficial (128))
　cerebral vein
4 Anteromedial (anterior
　internal (128)) frontal
　artery
5 Callosomarginal artery
6 Coronal suture
7 Anterior cerebral artery
8 Artery to precentral sulcus
　(Prerolandic artery (128))
9 Insular arteries
10 Frontal horn of lateral
　ventricle
11 Anterior vein of septum
　pellucidum
12 Internal cerebral vein
13 Third ventricle
14 Parietal bone
15 Temporo-occipital artery
　(128)
16 Lateral posterior choroid
　artery
17 Medial posterior choroid
　artery
18 Pineal gland (pineal body,
　epiphysis)
19 Great cerebral vein
　(Galen)
20 Choroid plexus in lateral
　ventricle
21 Medial occipital artery
22 Calcarine artery
23 Tentorium of cerebellum
24 Straight sinus
25 Lambdoidal suture
26 Occipital bone

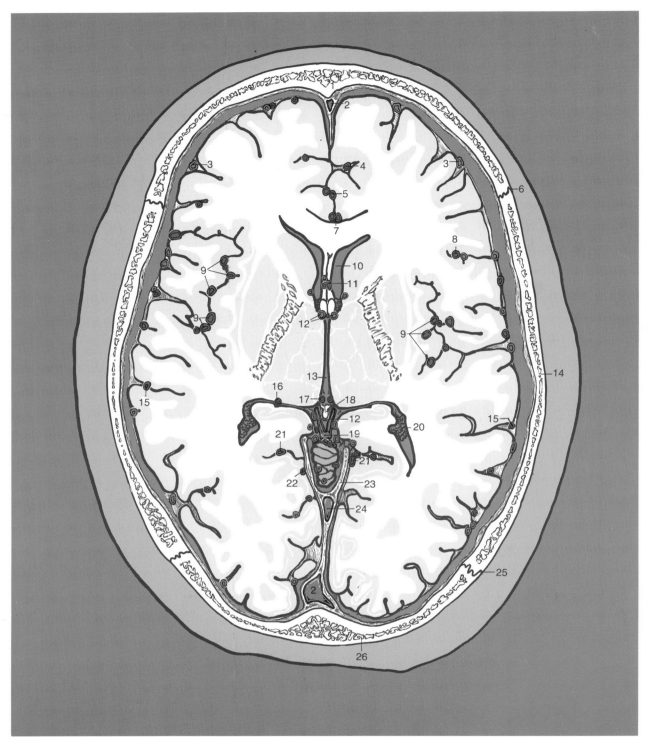

Fig. 12a　Cranial sectioning surface of the eighth slice. The pineal gland lies between the upper and lower surfaces of this slice. The internal cerebral veins cover the pineal gland. Only a small portion of its cranial surface can be seen. The sectioning plane runs through the lateral and third ventricles. The ridge of the tentorium of cerebellum is dissected. Bony structures and blood vessels.

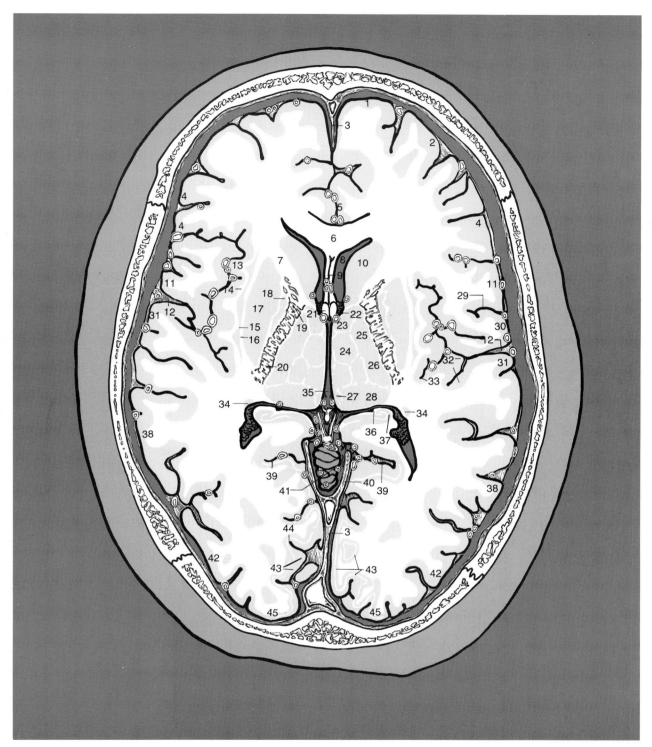

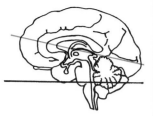

1 Superior frontal gyrus
2 Middle frontal gyrus
3 Cerebral falx
4 Inferior frontal gyrus
5 Cingulate gyrus
6 Corpus callosum
7 Anterior limb (crus) of internal capsule
8 Frontal horn of lateral ventricle
9 Cavum of septum pellucidum
10 Head of caudate nucleus
11 Precentral gyrus
12 Posterior branch of lateral sulcus
13 Insula (island of Reil)
14 Extreme capsule
15 Claustrum
16 External capsule
17 Putamen
18 Globus pallidus
19 Genu of internal capsule
20 Posterior limb (crus) of internal capsule
21 Fornix
22 Interventricular foramen (Monro)
23 Anterior nucleus of thalamus
24 Medial nucleus of thalamus
25 Ventral lateral nucleus of thalamus (nucleus ventrooralis (107))
26 Lateral posterior nucleus of thalamus
27 Habenular nuclei
28 Nuclei pulvinares
29 Central sulcus
√30 Postcentral gyrus
31 Superior temporal gyrus
32 Transverse temporal gyri (Heschl)
33 Circular sulcus of insula
34 Tail of caudate nucleus
35 Third ventricle
36 Fimbria of hippocampus
37 Hippocampus
38 Middle temporal gyrus
39 Parieto-occipital sulcus
40 Tentorium of cerebellum
41 Vermis of anterior lobe (from above)
42 Occipital gyri
43 Visual cortex
44 Calcarine sulcus
45 Occipital pole

Fig. 12b Cranial sectioning surface of the eighth slice. The sectioning plane passes through the insula, striatum (putamen and caudate nucleus), internal capsule, and thalamus. Lying caudal to the sectioning plane, and therefore not shown, are the superior colliculi, which are located between the third ventricle and the cerebellar vermis. Brain structures and meninges.

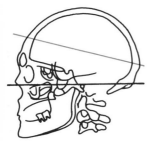

1 Frontal bone
2 Superior sagittal sinus
3 Superior (superficial (128)) cerebral vein
4 Mediomedial (middle internal (128)) frontal artery
5 Prefrontal artery
6 Callosomarginal artery
7 Coronal suture
8 Pericallosal artery
9 Artery to precentral sulcus (Prerolandic artery (128))
10 Insular arteries
11 Superior thalamostriate vein and stria terminalis
12 Superior choroidal vein
13 Central part of lateral ventricle
14 Artery to central sulcus (Rolandic artery (128))
15 Lateral posterior choroid artery
16 Collateral trigone and choroid plexus
17 Parietal artery
18 Parietal bone
19 Angular artery
20 Great cerebral vein (Galen)
21 Parieto-occipital artery
22 Straight sinus
23 Calcarine artery
24 Lambdoidal suture
25 Occipital bone

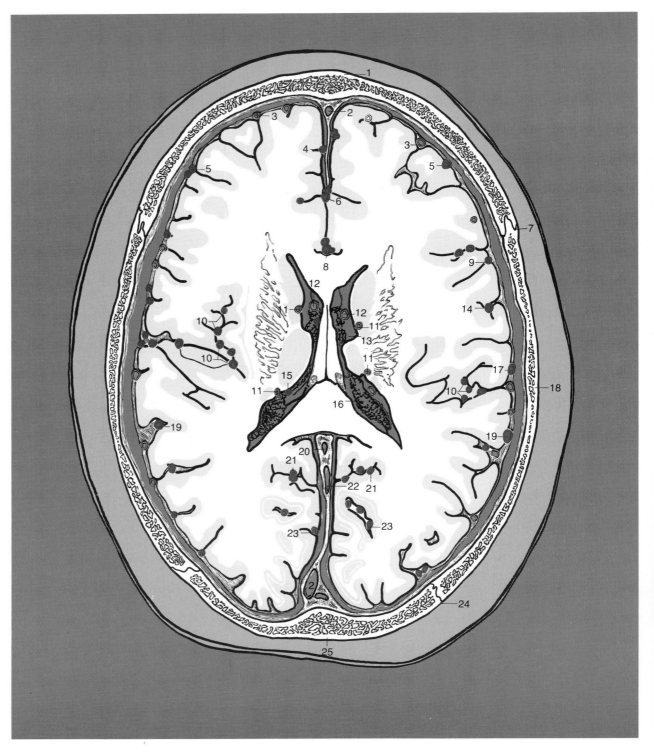

Fig. 13a　Cranial sectioning surface of the ninth slice. The sectioning plane passes through the central parts of the lateral ventricles (cella media) and lies just above the collateral trigone of the lateral ventricles. Bony structures and blood vessels.

Fig. 13b Cranial sectioning surface of the ninth slice. The sectioning plane divides the cerebral falx into a ventral and a dorsal part. The cranial portion of the insula is seen. The splenium of the corpus callosum lies between the collateral trigone of the right and left ventricles. Brain structures and meninges.

1 Superior frontal gyrus
2 Middle frontal gyrus
3 Cerebral falx
4 Cingulate sulcus
5 Cingulate gyrus
6 Frontal (minor) forceps
7 Inferior frontal gyrus
8 Trunk of corpus callosum
9 Precentral gyrus
10 Frontal horn of lateral ventricle
11 Central sulcus
12 Head of caudate nucleus
13 Claustrum
14 Insula (island of Reill)
15 Postcentral gyrus
16 Corona radiata
17 Posterior branch of lateral sulcus
18 Thalamus
19 Fornix
20 Superior temporal gyrus
21 Transverse temporal gyri (Heschl)
22 Tail of caudate nucleus
23 Splenium of corpus callosum
24 Occipital (major) forceps
25 Parieto-occipital sulcus
26 Cuneus
27 Occipital gyri
28 Visual cortex

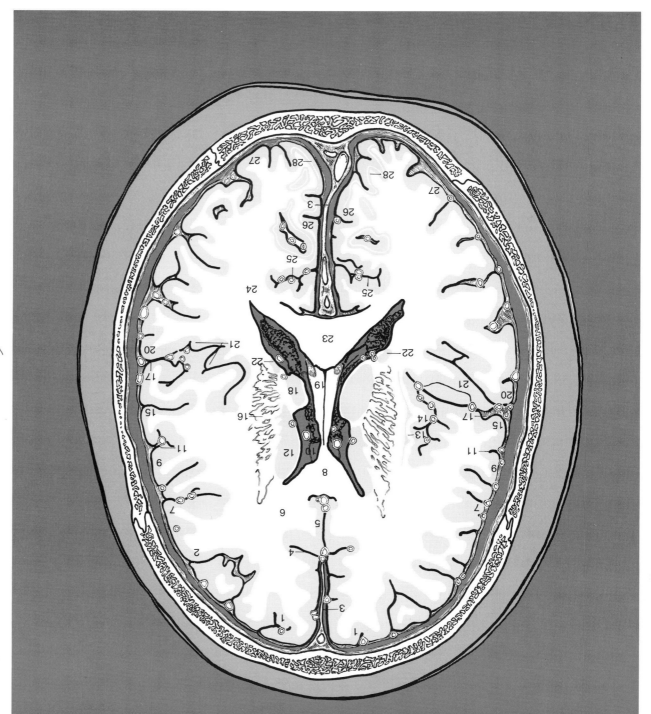

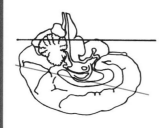

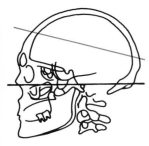

1 Frontal bone
2 Superior sagittal sinus
3 Superior (superficial (128))
   cerebral vein
4 Mediomedial (middle internal (128)) frontal artery
5 Prefrontal artery
6 Coronal suture
7 Callosomarginal artery
8 Artery to precentral sulcus
   (Prerolandic artery (128))
9 Artery to central sulcus
   (Rolandic artery (128))
10 Pericallosal artery
11 Parietal artery
12 Central part of lateral
   ventricle
13 Parietal bone
14 Inferior sagittal sinus
15 Angular artery
16 Parieto-occipital artery
17 Lambdoidal suture
18 Occipital bone

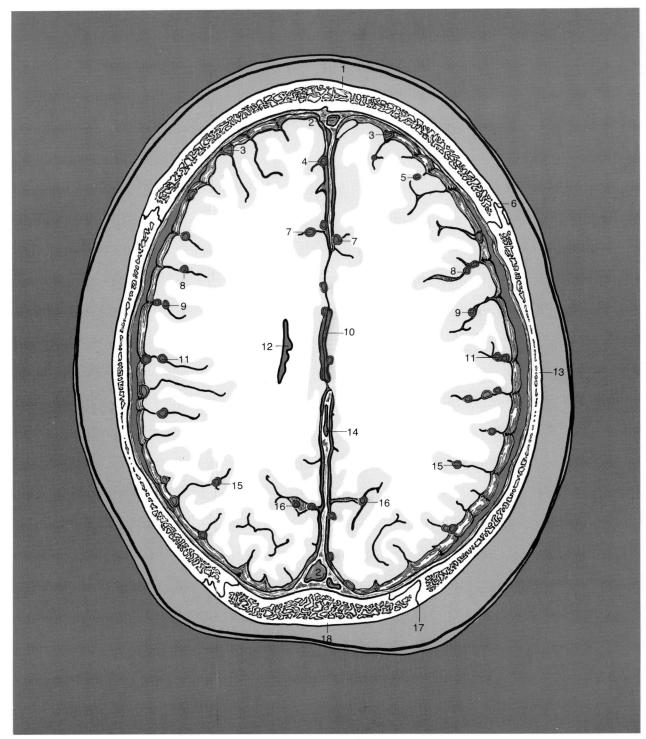

Fig. 14a   Cranial sectioning surface of the tenth slice.
The corpus callosum, which is not seen, forms the roof
of the cella media. On the left side the lateral ventricle is
cut open. Bony structures and blood vessels.

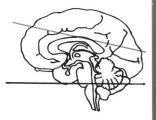

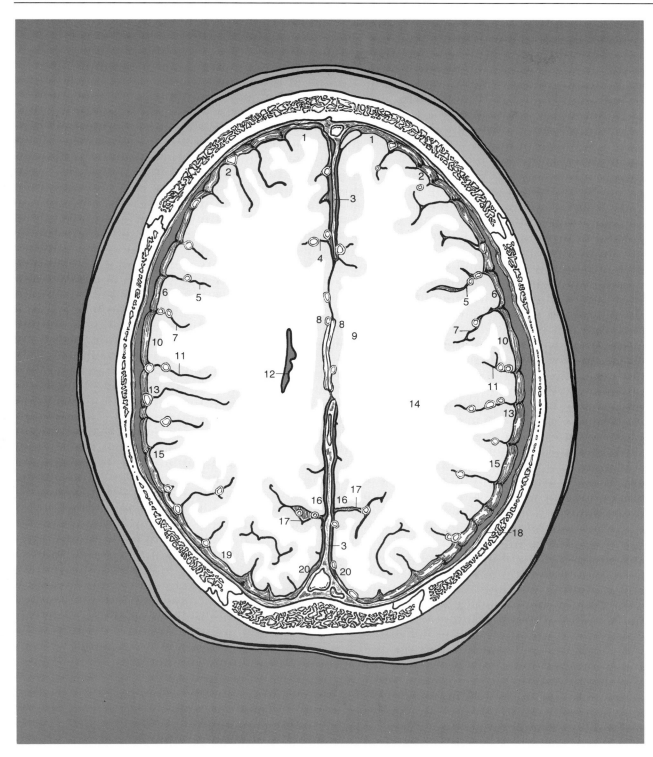

1 Superior frontal gyrus
2 Middle frontal gyrus
3 Cerebral falx
4 Cingulate sulcus
5 Precentral sulcus
6 Precentral gyrus
7 Central sulcus
8 Cingulate gyrus
9 Cingulum
10 Postcentral gyrus
11 Postcentral sulcus
12 Central part of lateral ventricle
13 Supramarginal gyrus
14 Semioval center
15 Angular gyrus
16 Precuneus
17 Parieto-occipital sulcus
18 Dura mater
19 Occipital gyri
20 Cuneus

Fig. 14b   Cranial sectioning surface of the tenth slice. The sectioning plane divides the cerebral falx into a ventral and a dorsal part. Between these two parts lies the supracommissural portion of the cingulate gyrus which covers the corpus callosum. Brain structures and meninges.

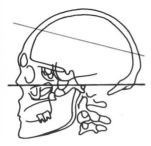

1 Frontal bone
2 Superior sagittal sinus
3 Superior (superficial (128))
   cerebral vein
4 Mediomedial (middle internal (128)) frontal artery
5 Prefrontal artery
6 Coronal suture
7 Callosomarginal artery
8 Artery to precentral sulcus
   (Prerolandic artery (128))
9 Artery to central sulcus
   (Rolandic artery (128))
10 Paracentral artery
11 Parietal bone
12 Parietal artery
13 Precuneal artery
14 Angular artery
15 Parieto-occipital artery
16 Occipital bone
17 Lambdoidal suture

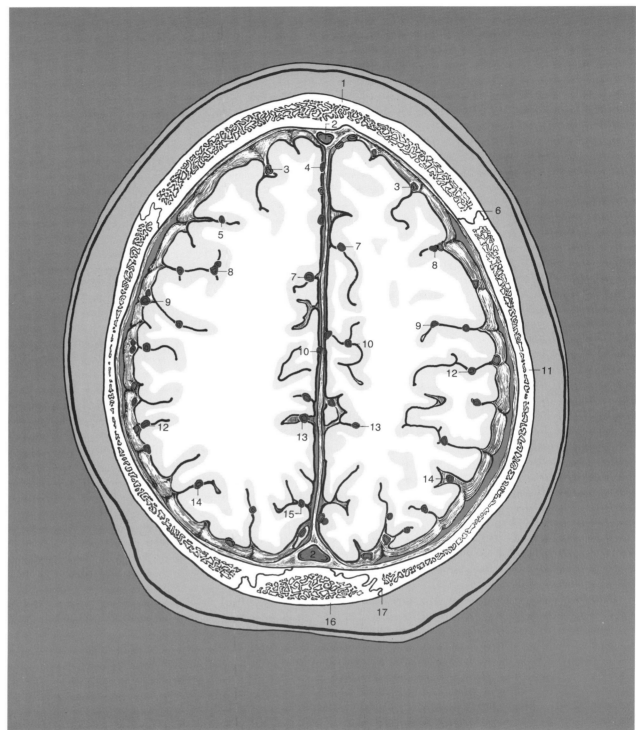

Fig. 15a Cranial sectioning surface of the eleventh
slice. This section lies in a supraventricular position.
Bony structures and blood vessels.

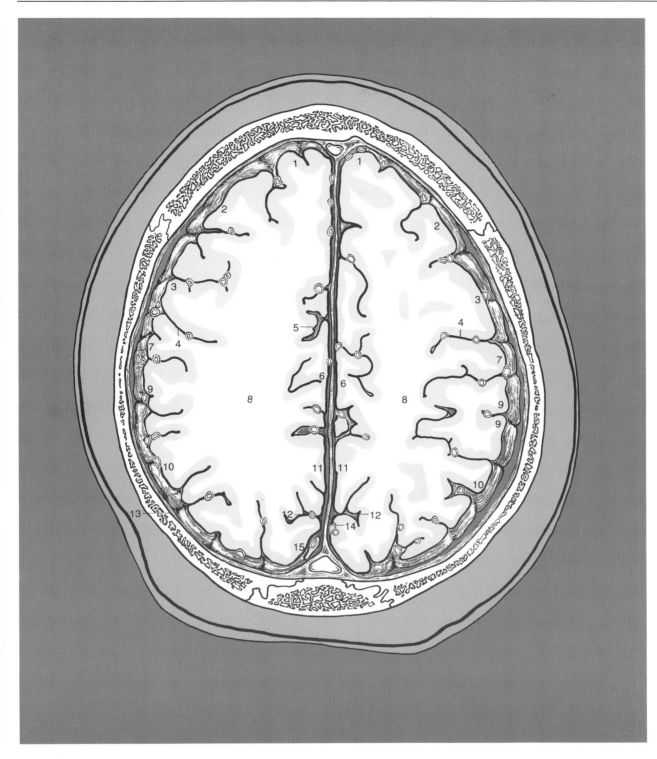

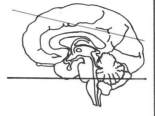

1 Superior frontal gyrus
2 Middle frontal gyrus
3 Precentral gyrus
4 Central sulcus
5 Cingulate sulcus
6 Cingulate gyrus
7 Postcentral gyrus
8 Semioval center
9 Supramarginal gyrus
10 Angular gyrus
11 Precuneus
12 Parieto-occipital sulcus
13 Dura mater
14 Cerebral falx
15 Cuneus

Fig. 15b Cranial sectioning surface of the eleventh slice. The sectioning plane cuts the cingulate gyrus tangentially. The cerebral falx separates the right and left hemispheres. The caudal edge of the cerebral falx is located in the middle of the section and, therefore, is not visible. Brain structures and meninges.

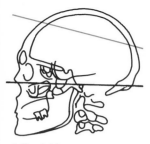

1 Frontal bone
2 Superior sagittal sinus
3 Posteromedial (posterior internal (128)) frontal artery
4 Superior (superficial (128)) cerebral vein
5 Coronal suture
6 Parietal bone
7 Paracentral artery
8 Precuneal artery
9 Sagittal suture
10 Scalp (epicranium)
11 Skin of the head

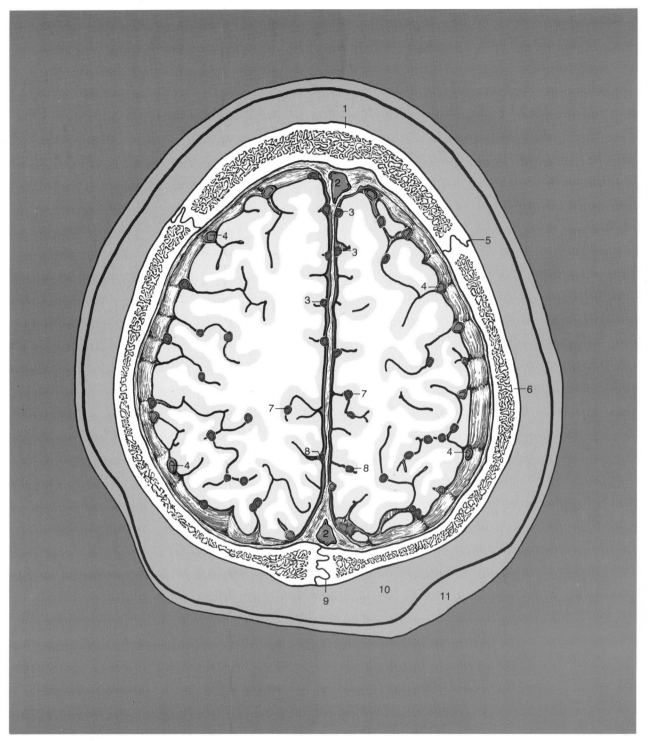

Fig. 16a Cranial sectioning surface of the twelfth slice. This section lies in a supraventricular position. Bony structures and blood vessels.

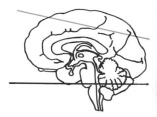

1 Superior frontal gyrus
2 Middle frontal gyrus
3 Precentral sulcus
4 Precentral gyrus
5 Central sulcus
6 Postcentral gyrus
7 Semioval center
8 Paracentral lobule
9 Superior parietal lobule
10 Cerebral falx
11 Precuneus
12 Parieto-occipital sulcus
13 Dura mater

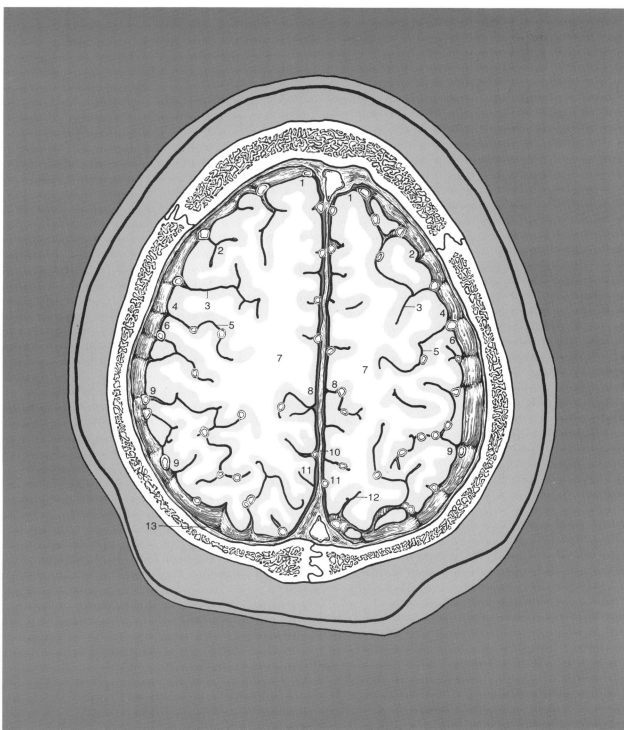

Fig. 16b Cranial sectioning surface of the twelfth slice. The cerebral falx extends straight through the entire section separating the left from the right hemisphere. This section lies above the cingulate gyrus. Brain structures and meninges.

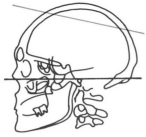

1 Frontal bone
2 Superior sagittal sinus
3 Coronal suture
4 Posteromedial (posterior internal (128)) frontal artery
5 Superior (superficial (128)) cerebral vein
6 Parietal bone
7 Paracentral artery
8 Precuneal artery
9 Sagittal suture

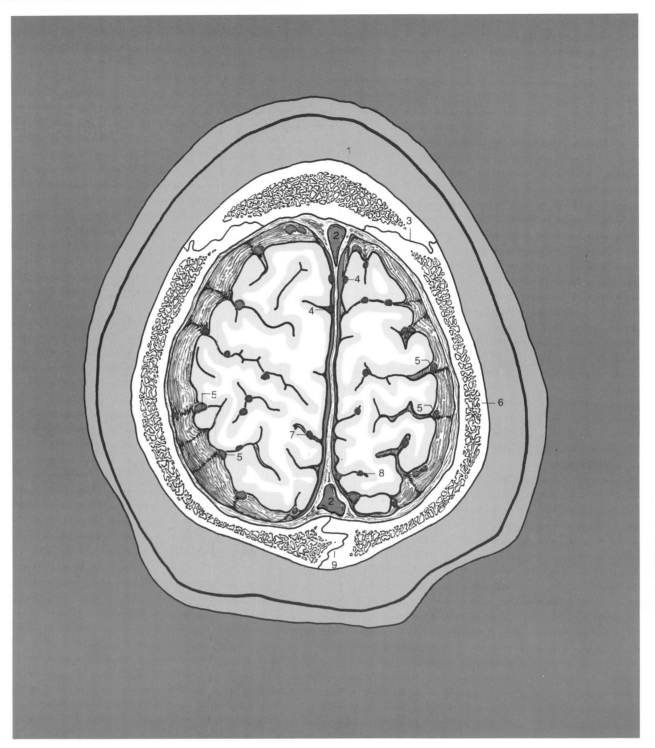

Fig. 17a Cranial sectioning surface of the thirteenth slice. This section lies in a supraventricular position. Bony structures and blood vessels

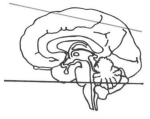

1 Superior frontal gyrus
2 Precentral sulcus
3 Precentral gyrus
4 Central sulcus
5 Postcentral gyrus
6 Paracentral lobule
7 Cerebral falx
8 Dura mater
9 Superior parietal lobule
10 Precuneus

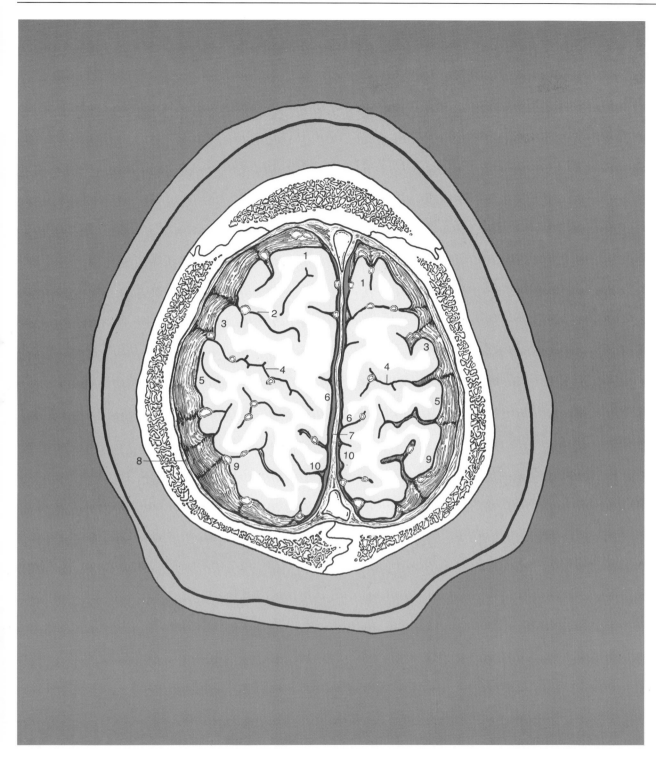

Fig. 17b Cranial sectioning surface of the thirteenth slice. The central sulcus separates the frontal from the parietal lobe. Brain structures and meninges.

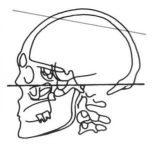

1 Frontal bone
2 Bregma
3 Coronal suture
4 Superior (superficial (128))
  cerebral vein
5 Superior sagittal sinus
6 Parietal bone
7 Sagittal suture
8 Scalp (epicranium)
9 Skin of the head

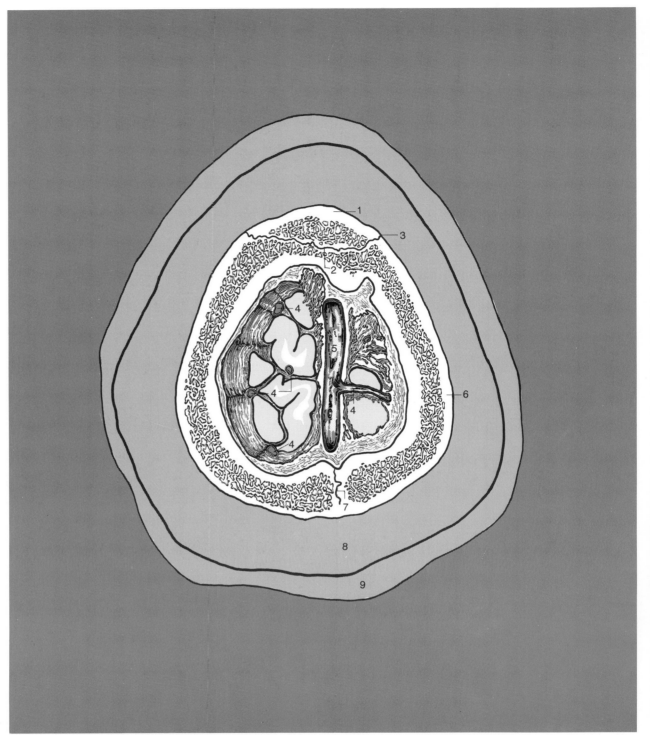

Fig. 18a Cranial sectioning surface of the fourteenth slice. This section is supraventricular just beneath the top of the skullcap. Bony structures and blood vessels.

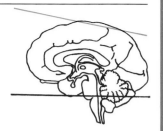

1 Precentral gyrus
2 Central sulcus
3 Postcentral gyrus
4 Dura mater

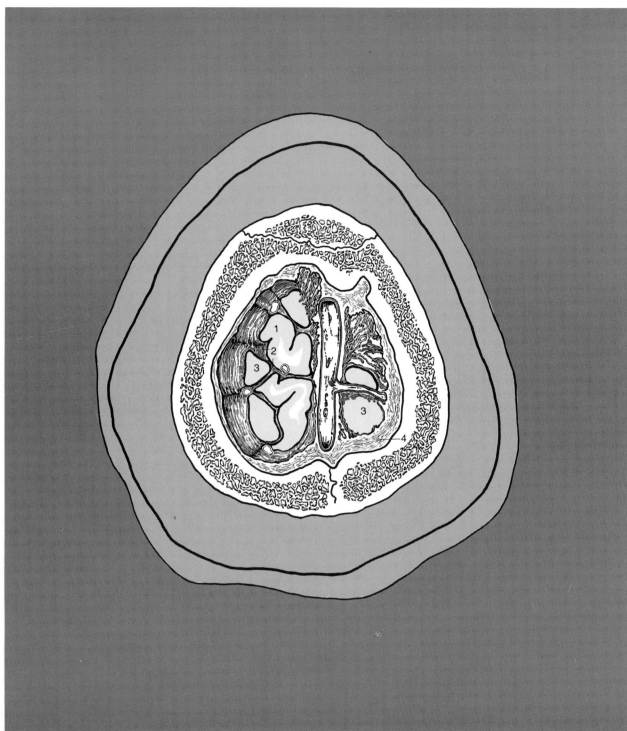

Fig. 18b Cranial sectioning surface of the fourteenth slice. The central sulcus lies approximately 5 cm dorsal of the bregma. Brain structures and meninges.

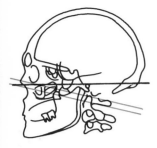

1 Nasal bone
2 Maxilla
3 Nasal septum
4 Infraorbital canal
5 Zygomatic bone
6 Maxillary sinus
7 Palatine bone
8 Lateral lamina of pterygoid
  process
9 Mandible
10 Anterior arch of atlas
11 Styloid process
12 Dens of axis
13 Transverse foramen of
   atlas
14 Lateral mass of atlas
15 Vertebral canal
16 Auricle (pinna)
17 Posterior arch of atlas

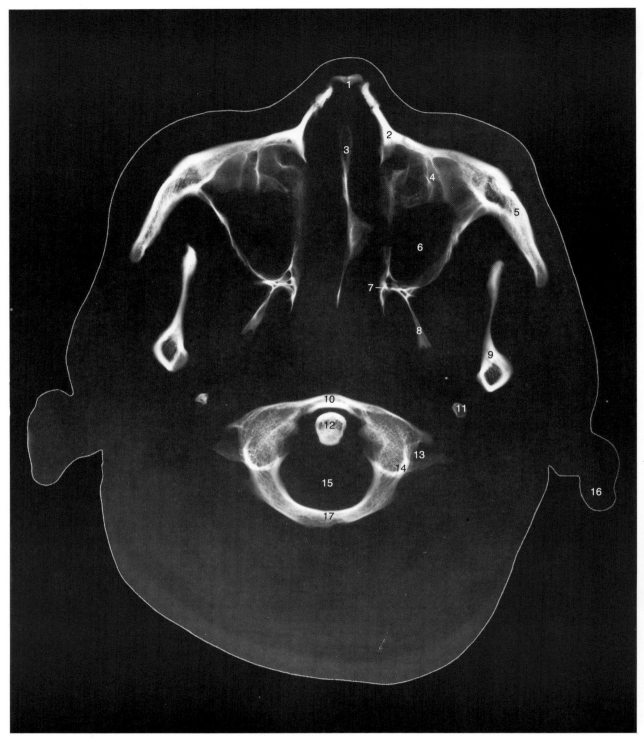

Fig. 19   X-ray of the first slice. The outer border of the head has been added. Guideline structures include the maxillary sinuses, atlas, and dens of axis.

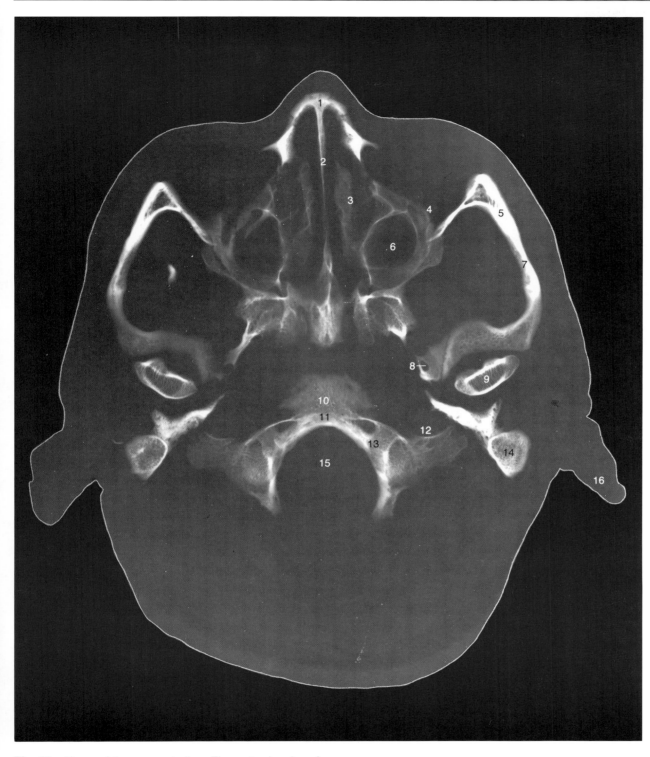

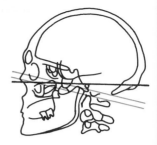

1 Nasal bone
2 Nasal septum
3 Ethmoidal cells (sinus)
4 Orbit
5 Zygomatic bone
6 Maxillary sinus
7 Zygomatic arch
8 Spinous foramen
9 Mandible
10 Basilar part of occipital bone
11 Basion
12 Jugular foramen
13 Hypoglossal canal
14 Mastoid process
15 Foramen magnum
16 Auricle (pinna)

Fig. 20 X-ray of the second slice. The outer border of the head has been added. Bony guideline structures include the nasal bone, nasal septum, and foramen magnum.

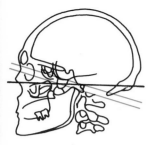

1 Ethmoidal cells (sinus)
2 Orbit
3 Zygomatic bone
4 Ethmoid bone
5 Foramen rotundum
6 Sphenoid sinus
7 Sphenoid bone, floor of
   middle cranial fossa
8 Oval foramen
9 Temporal bone
10 Foramen lacerum
11 Spinous foramen
12 Clivus
13 Head of mandible
14 Carotid canal
15 External acoustic (auditory) meatus
16 Jugular foramen
17 Facial canal
18 Mastoid process
19 Occipital bone, floor of
   posterior cranial fossa

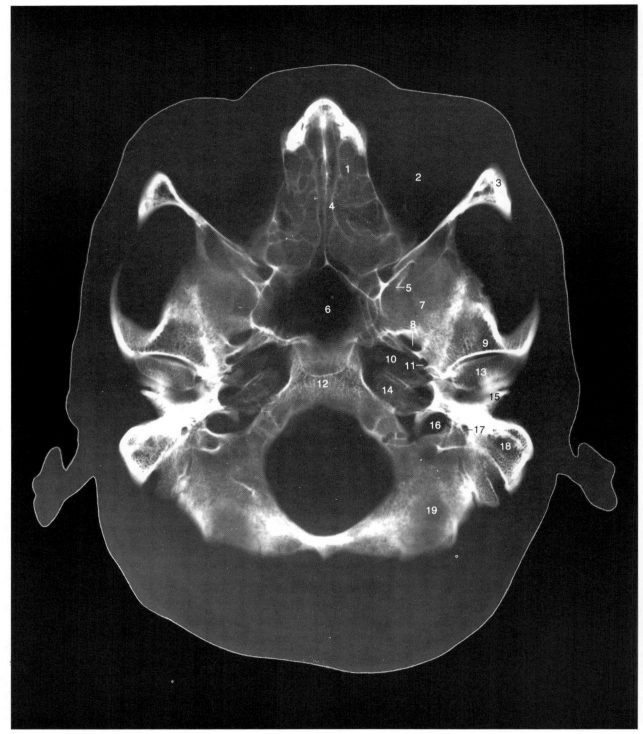

Fig. 21 X-ray of the third slice. The medial and lateral walls of the orbits are shown. The sphenoid bone forms the floor of the middle cranial fossa. The occipital bone encloses the posterior cranial fossa. The openings for the internal carotid arteries, internal jugular veins, middle meningeal arteries, as well as those for cranial nerves V/2, V/3, VII, IX, X, XI are shown.

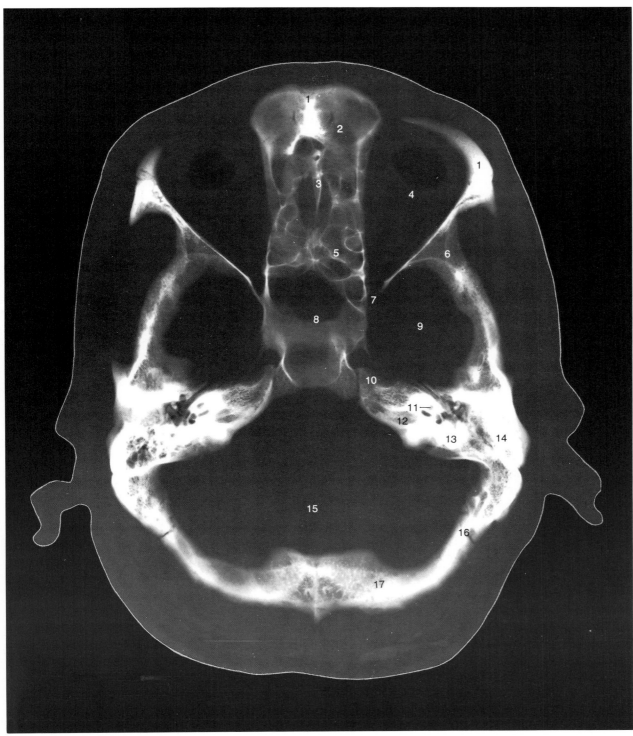

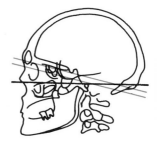

1 Frontal bone
2 Floor of frontal sinus
3 Crista galli
4 Orbit
5 Ethmoidal cells (sinus)
6 Sphenoid bone
7 Superior orbital fissure
8 Sphenoid sinus
9 Middle cranial fossa
10 Apex of petrous part of
   temporal bone
11 Cochlea
12 Internal acoustic (auditory)
   meatus
13 Petrous part of temporal
   bone
14 Temporal bone
15 Posterior cranial fossa
16 Lambdoidal suture
17 Occipital bone

Fig. 22 X-ray of the fourth slice, showing the upper portion of the orbits, sphenoid sinus, middle cranial fossa, petrous bones, and posterior cranial fossa.

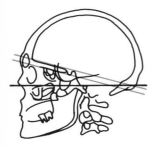

1 Frontal bone
2 Frontal sinus
3 Roof of orbit
4 Anterior cranial fossa
5 Sphenoid bone
6 Optic canal
7 Anterior clinoid process
8 Sella turcica (pituitary
  fossa)
9 Middle cranial fossa
10 Posterior clinoid process
11 Dorsum sellae
12 Anterior semicircular canal
13 Posterior semicircular
   canal
14 Temporal bone
15 Posterior cranial fossa
16 Lambdoidal suture
17 Internal occipital protuberance
18 Occipital bone
19 External occipital protuberance (inion)

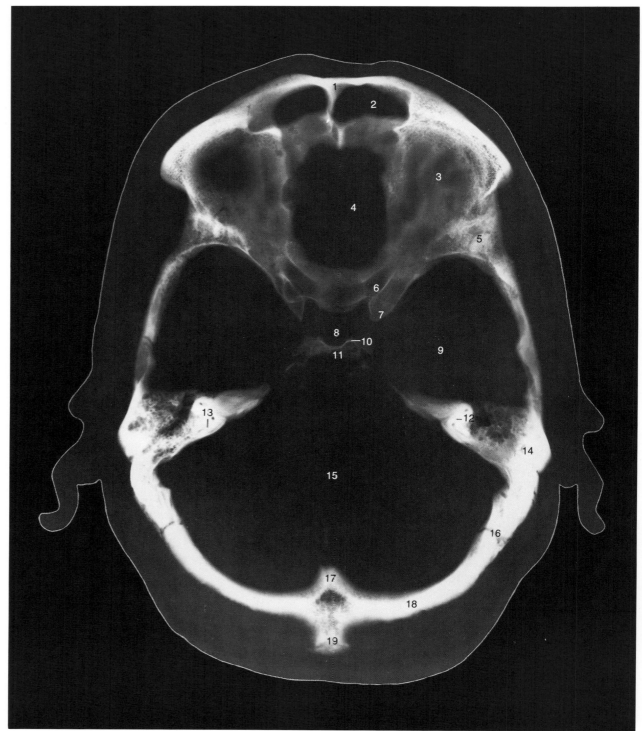

Fig. 23   X-ray of the fifth slice showing the floor of the anterior cranial fossa, anterior clinoid processes, dorsum sellae, and cranial portion of the petrous bones.

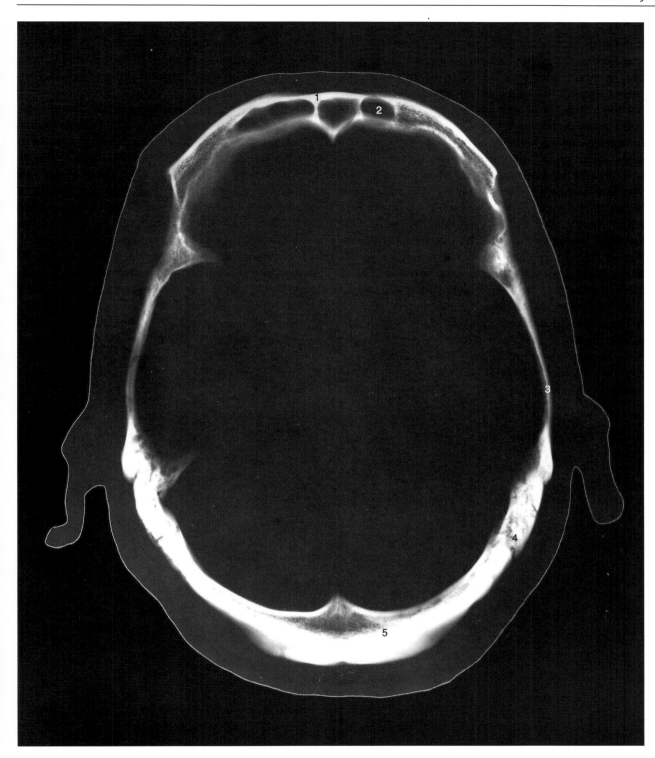

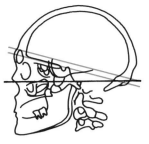

1 Frontal bone
2 Frontal sinus
3 Temporal bone
4 Lambdoidal suture
5 Occipital bone

Fig. 24 X-ray of the sixth slice. The skull forms an oval bony ring. Its inner processes, marking the borders of the anterior, middle, and posterior cranial fossae, are seen more clearly to the left.

As seen in the parallel canthomeatal planes, the serial cross sections of the bones at the skull base and craniocervical junction appear as more complicated images when compared to those of the skullcap. Depending on the shape of the head, the superior portion of the skull appears in cross sections as a bony, more or less oval ring (Figs. 10a–18a).

In sections through the craniocervical junction, CT scans show great variability when higher cervical vertebrae or intervertebral spaces are cut (Fig. 5a). The first cervical vertebra, the atlas, is characterized by the anterior and posterior arches, an absent vertebral body, and laterally positioned transverse foramina through which the vertebral arteries ascend. These structures are better visualized in the X-ray of the 1 cm thick section (Fig. 19). The second cervical vertebra, the axis, is easily identified by its tooth-like process, the dens.

In Figure 6a, the sectioning plane lies at a slight angle to the foramen magnum, dissecting ventrally the basal portion of the occipital bone and ventrolaterally the hypoglossal canal. The dorsal part of the sectioning plane is located in a caudal position close to the foramen magnum (Fig. 20).

The topography of the posterior, middle, and anterior cranial fossae is best clarified on the skull itself. "Hands-on" examination of the skull allows to understand the spatial relationships of these structures most easily. Simply by studying illustrations of the internal cranial base in anatomic atlases, an incorrect idea of the arrangement of these fossae may result. In an atlas, the fossae frequently appear to lie on the same horizontal plane. In reality, the three cranial fossae build three terraces, each set about 2.5 cm above or below the other (168). The floor of the middle cranial fossa lies approximately in Reid's base plane (Fig. 2 DH) (79). The floor of the posterior fossa is about 2.5 cm lower and the anterior fossa 2.5 cm higher than the middle cranial fossa. Knowledge of such simple spatial relationships is very useful when examining cross-sectional images made in parallel canthomeatal planes. On the average, the canthomeatal plane is tilted 19° to Reid's base line (168). The canthomeatal plane lies within the head slice (Fig. 7a). The sectioning plane lies in the caudal third of the posterior cranial fossa and extends along the floor of the middle fossa. The anterior fossa lies cranial to the sectioning plane, and hence is not shown in the illustrations. The X-ray of this slice shows the jugular foramen in the posterior fossa and the spinous, oval, and round foramina in the middle cranial fossa (Fig. 21).

In the next slice (Figs. 8a and 22), the skull encloses the posterior and middle cranial fossae in the form of two forceps. The opening of the internal acoustic (auditory) meatus is found in the posterior cranial fossa (Fig. 8a.15). The superior orbital fissure joins the middle cranial fossa with the orbit (Figs. 8a.6 and 22.7). In the middle of Figure 8a the dorsum sellae has been partially dissected (Fig. 8a.11). The cribriform plate is shown as a part of the anterior cranial fossa. Resting on the cribriform plate is the olfactory bulb (Fig. 8b.3).

In the fifth slice, the sectioning plane dissects the tentorium of cerebellum (Fig. 9a.17). The infratentorial compartment appears to decrease gradually in size in the subsequent cranial slices until it finally reaches the ridge of the tentorium. The X-ray of this slice shows the optic canal (Fig. 23.6) which forms a connection between the orbit and the middle cranial fossa. The roof of the orbit can be seen in the anterior cranial fossa (Figs. 9a.4 and 23.3).

In the subsequent slice (Figs. 10a and 24) and in all further slices, the bony outline of the skull appears as an oval ring. The infratentorial compartment forms a smaller portion of these illustrations than the supratentorial compartment. The border between the two compartments is marked by the tentorium of cerebellum (Fig. 10a.17).

3.2 Cerebrospinal Fluid Containing Spaces (Figs. 25–27)

Due to its almost identical specific gravity with the cerebrospinal fluid, the brain floats in its protective jacket of cerebrospinal fluid (CSF) (321). CSF is present throughout the ventricular system and the subarachnoid space. The subarachnoid space, which lies between the pia mater and the more external located arachnoid, holds approximately 25–50 ml of CSF (168, 264). The arachnoid lies direct on the dura mater, a tough fibrous membrane. Except when enlarged or in the area of cisterns, CT scans of living patients do not demonstrate the subarachnoid space. Due to the alcohol-formalin fixation, the subarachnoid spaces of our anatomical preparations are artificially enlarged.

Expansions of the CSF jacket in the subarachnoid space are referred to as cisterns. The cisterna magna (cerebellomedullary cistern) fills the space between the medulla oblongata, the roof of the fourth ventricle, and the inferior surface of the cerebellum. It is approximately 3 cm wide and in the sagittal plane up to 2 cm deep. In the median plane indentations are present, as the cistern follows the highly variable surface of the cerebellar falx. This is the cistern entered during suboccipital (cisternal) puncture.

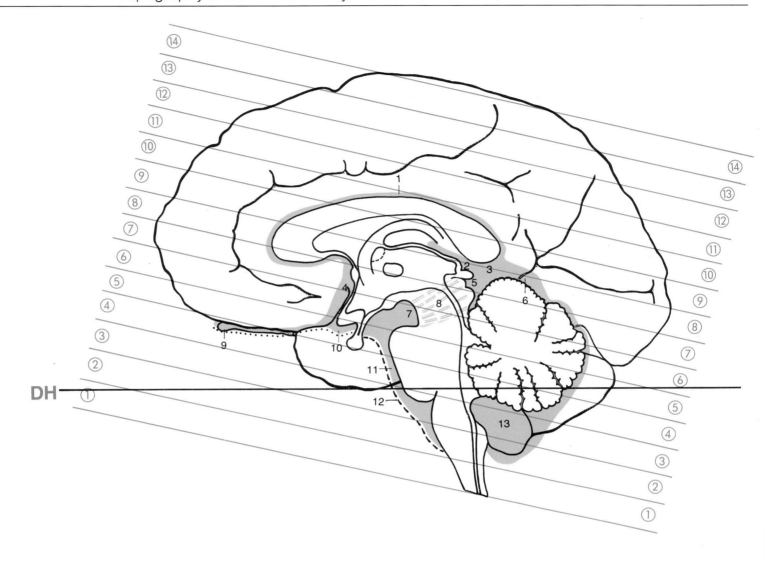

Fig. 25   Medial view of the external CSF spaces. The ambient cistern laterally encloses the cerebral peduncle. This cistern is therefore indicated with a broken blue line. According to (247).

1 Pericallosal cistern
2 Cistern of transverse fissure (168) (cistern of velum interpositum (325))
3 Cistern of great cerebral vein (Galen)
4 Cistern of lamina terminalis
5 Cistern of tectal lamina (quadrigeminal cistern (325))
6 Superior cerebellar cistern

7 Interpeduncular cistern
8 Ambient cistern
9 Anterior basal cistern (168) (dotted line)
10 Chiasmatic cistern
11 Pontine cistern
12 Posterior basal cistern (167) (interrupted line)
13 Cisterna magna (cerebellomedullary cistern)

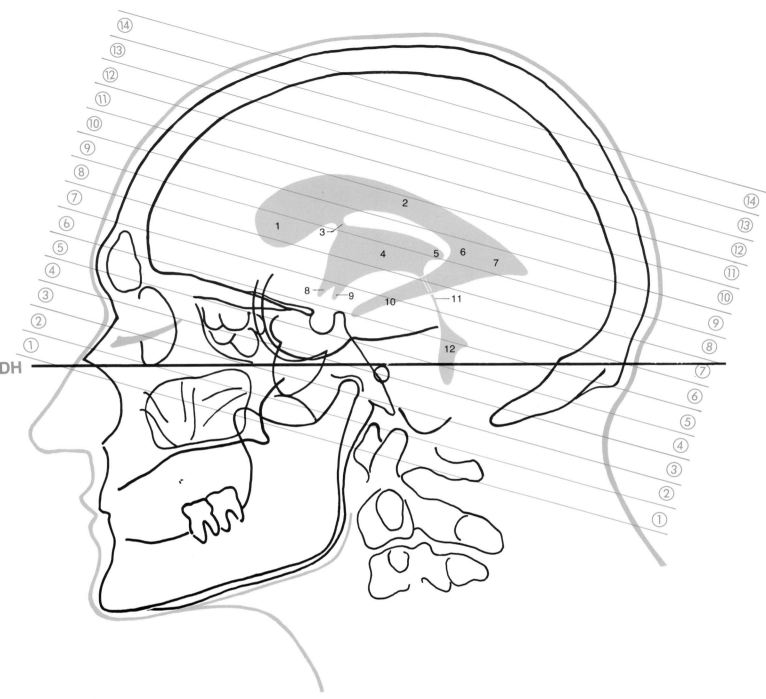

Fig. 26 Lateral view of the ventricular system derived from an X-ray of the head of a 44-year-old male (see Figs. 1a, 2, 3, 4).
DH = Reid's base line = "Deutsche Horizontale".

1 Frontal (anterior) horn
2 Central part (cella media)
3 Interventricular foramen
  (Monro)
4 Third ventricle
5 Suprapineal recess
6 Collateral trigone
7 Occipital (posterior) horn
8 Optic recess
9 Infundibular recess
10 Temporal (inferior) horn
11 Aqueduct
12 Fourth ventricle

1 Posterior basal cistern
   (167)
2 Cisterna magna (cerebellomedullary cistern)
3 Anterior basal cistern (168)
4 Pontine cistern
5 Trigeminal cistern
6 Cerebellopontine (angle)
   cistern (325)
7 Fourth ventricle
8 Cistern of vallecula cerebri
   (167)
9 Suprasellar cistern (pentagon)
10 Lateral ventricle

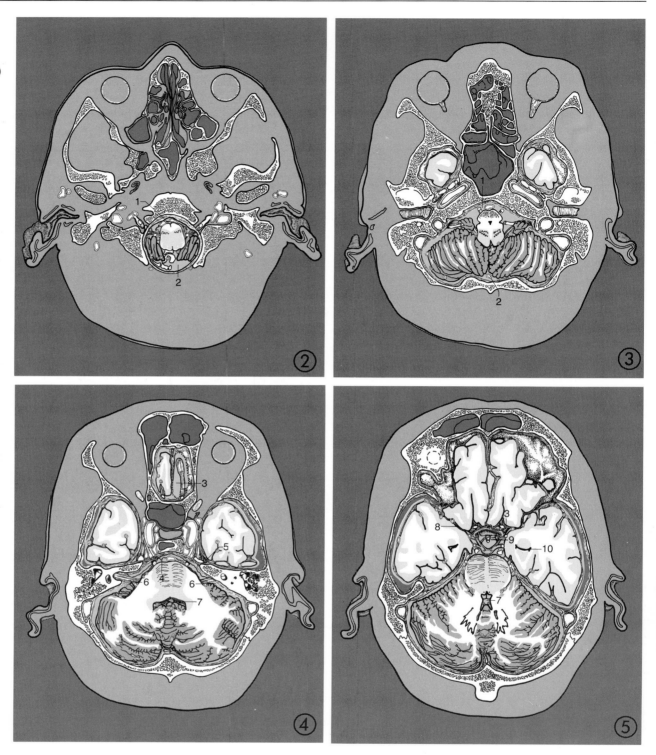

Fig. 27 Serial illustrations of the intracranial CSF spaces. The encircled number indicates the number of the respective slice (see Figs. 1a, 2, 3, 4, 25, 26).

8 Cistern of vallecula cerebri (167)
10 Lateral ventricle
11 Interhemispheric cistern
12 Cistern of lamina terminalis
13 Cistern of lateral (Sylvian) fissure (insular cistern)
14 Third ventricle
15 Ambient cistern
16 Transition of aqueduct into the fourth ventricle
17 Pericallosal cistern
18 Aqueduct
19 Cistern of tectal lamina (quadrigeminal cistern (325))
20 Superior cerebellar cistern
21 Cistern of great cerebral vein (Galen)

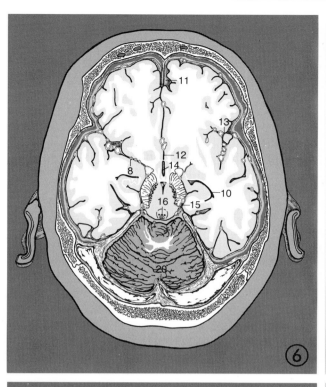

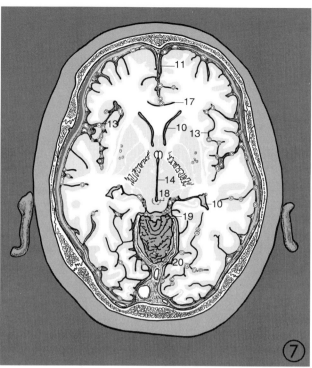

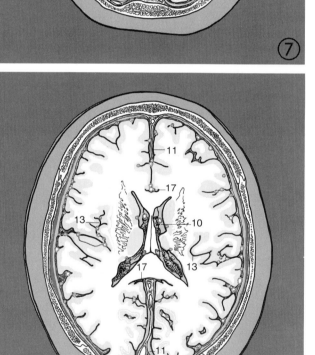

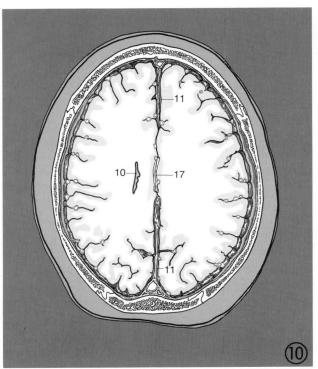

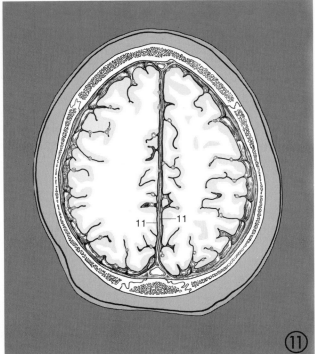

Fig. 27

The posterior and anterior basal cisterns are enlarged cavities of the subarachnoid space. These basal cisterns are located between the base of the brain and the skull base and extend from the foramen magnum to the crista galli on the anterior edge of the anterior cranial fossa. The posterior and anterior basal cisterns are separated by the dorsum sellae (168). The pontine cistern and the paired cerebellopontine (angle) cisterns are lying in the posterior cranial fossa. The pontine cistern is located between clivus and pons. The two cerebellopontine cisterns lie in the cerebellopontine angle. The flocculus of the cerebellum extends laterally into each cerebellopontine cistern. The lateral recess of the fourth ventricle also opens into these cisterns through the lateral apertures (Luschka).

The lateral apertures (Luschka) are easily identified by "Bochdalek's bouquet". The latter is a part of the choroid plexus of the fourth ventricle protruding through the paired lateral apertures (Luschka). The superior cerebellar cistern is found between the tentorium and the superior surface of the cerebellum. The rostral portion of the posterior basal cistern is formed by the interpeduncular cistern. Originating in the similarly named fossa, the interpeduncular cistern contains the third cranial nerve, the terminal bifurcation of the basilar artery (Fig. 9a.14), as well as the origin of the superior cerebellar arteries and the posterior cerebral arteries (Fig. 9a.13).

The ambient cistern lies at the border between the posterior and middle cranial fossae and is connected to the interpeduncular cistern. The ambient cistern encloses the lateral surfaces of the cerebral peduncles and forms a fluid jacket around the tentorial notch (incisura) against the sharp edge of the tentorium of cerebellum. The ambient cistern continues dorsally as the cistern of the tectal lamina (quadrigeminal cistern) and the cistern of the great cerebral vein (Galen), and rostrally as the cistern of the vallecula cerebri. Furthermore, the ambient cistern is connected with the unpaired pericallosal cistern and the paired interhemispheric cisterns. The ambient cistern contains three blood vessels with a dorsal direction of flow: the posterior cerebral artery, the superior cerebellar artery, and the basal vein (Rosenthal). The ambient cistern also contains the trochlear nerve that sends efferent signals in a ventral direction.

The trigeminal cistern opens into the cerebellopontine cistern. The flat appendix of the trigeminal cistern (Fig. 27.5) lies on the petrous portion of the temporal bone and sphenoid bone in the middle cranial fossa and houses the root of the fifth cranial nerve together with the trigeminal (Gasserian) ganglion.

The anterior basal cistern reaches from the dorsum sellae to the anterior edge of the anterior cranial fossa. This cistern borders on the mamillary bodies, infundibulum, optic chiasm, optic tracts, olfactory bulbs and tracts, and the base of the frontal lobes. One part of this cistern, the chiasmatic cistern, encloses the optic chiasm. The anterior basal cistern continues dorsally as the interpeduncular cistern. Hilal (120) introduced the term "pentagon"

(Fig. 27.9) meaning the suprasellar cistern. The cerebral arterial circle (circle of Willis) and its central branches lie in the pentagon.

The anterior basal cistern continues laterally through the cistern of the vallecula cerebri to the cistern of the lateral (Sylvian) fissure. The cistern of the vallecula cerebri is the CSF filled space between the posterior edge of the lesser wing of the sphenoid bone and the anterior perforated substance. The first segment of the middle cerebral artery is located here. The cistern of the lateral (Sylvian) fissure (Fig. 27.13) forms the space between the insula and the opercular portion of the frontal, parietal, and temporal lobes (18). Therefore, this space is also referred to as the insular cistern. The branches of the middle cerebral artery, the insular arteries, are found here.

The cistern of the transverse fissure (168) (cistern of the velum interpositum) (Fig. 25.2) is a fluid accumulation located in the fissure between the corpus callosum and the roof of the third ventricle including the thalamus. In other words, it lies between telencephalon and diencephalon; this fissure was previously known as the telodiencephalic fissure. The cistern of the transverse fissure extends rostrally toward the interventricular foramen (Monro) (Fig. 12b.22). It is 2.5 cm long in sagittal direction and has a transverse diameter of 4 cm. It contains the internal cerebral veins (Fig. 12a.12) and a portion of the posterior choroid arteries (Figs. 12a.16 and 12a.17).

The cistern of the transverse fissure continues as the cistern of the great cerebral vein (Galen), the pericallosal and interhemispheric cisterns. The pericallosal cistern is the unpaired CSF filled space between the corpus callosum and the inferior free edge of the cerebral falx. The interhemispheric cisterns are the paired fluid spaces between the cerebral falx and the medial surfaces of the cerebral hemispheres.

The cistern of the lamina terminalis connects the chiasmatic cistern with the pericallosal cistern. The latter encloses the corpus callosum.

The internal CSF containing spaces are the four ventricles with their connections. Volume and shape of these spaces vary greatly even among healthy individuals. The average ventricular volume of an extracranially fixed adult brain is approximately 20 ml, ranging from 7 to 57 ml (151, 174). According to CT examinations of healthy brains, the volume lies between 15 and 46 ml, the average being 31 ml (30). The fourth ventricle is connected by three openings to the subarachnoid space: at the obex through the unpaired median aperture (Magendie) and laterally at the medulla oblongata, next to the seventh cranial nerve, through the paired lateral apertures (Luschka). The fourth ventricle is shaped like a small tent; its floor being the rhomboid fossa and the roof being the two medullary vela, the cerebellar peduncles, and the cerebellum. The rostral part of the roof is formed by the superior medullary velum and the caudal portion by the inferior medullary velum. The choroid plexus of the fourth ventricle is attached to the inferior medullary velum. It is suspended on a sheet of connective tissue, forming the dorsal closure of the fourth ventricle.

The aqueduct (approximately 15 mm long) is located in the midbrain (Figs. 10b.33 and 11a.17). It curves slightly ventrally, connecting the fourth ventricle with the third.

The third ventricle is an unpaired slit-shaped cavity located in the median plane. Its walls are formed from its dorsal to basal portion by the epithalamus, thalamus, and hypothalamus. In 75% of the brains examined, an intermediate mass, the interthalamic adhesion could be demonstrated between the right and left thalamus. The lamina terminalis forms the rostral border of the third ventricle (Fig. 10b.16). In the area near the hypothalamic sulcus, a groove for the anterior commissure can be found. Near the hypothalamus, two additional appendices can be seen: the optic recess leading toward the optic chiasm and the infundibular recess directed toward the pituitary stalk (Figs. 26.8 and 26.9).

The choroid plexus appears as a canopy in the third ventricle above the interventricular foramen (Monro). Connected to the choroid plexus is a thin ependymal lining, the tela choroidea. It stretches between the medullary striae of the thalamus and forms an appendix above the pineal gland, the suprapineal recess. A few millimeters below the suprapineal recess is a small niche, the pineal recess. Located above the pineal and below the suprapineal recess is the habenular commissure. Underneath the pineal recess the posterior commissure is found, below which the aqueduct opens into the third ventricle (169).

The two lateral ventricles take the form of two ram horn-shaped cavities in the telencephalon. They are linked to each other and to the third ventricle by the interventricular foramina. In accordance with the four lobes of the telencephalon, the lateral ventricle is divided into four parts:

1. Frontal or anterior horn, located in the frontal lobe (Figs. 11b.7, 12b.8, 13b.10)
2. Central part, located in the parietal lobe (Figs. 13a.13 and 14b.12)
3. Occipital or posterior horn, located in the occipital lobe (it lies within the ninth slice and, hence, is not visible)
4. Temporal or inferior horn, located in the temporal lobe (Figs. 9b.13 and 10b.31).

The frontal horn forms the rostral pole of the lateral ventricle and reaches the interventricular foramen (Fig. 12b.22). The frontal horn is bordered medially by the septum pellucidum and laterally by the head of the caudate nucleus. The radiation of the corpus callosum forms its roof.

The central part of the lateral ventricle is narrow due to the protruding thalamus and is referred to as "thalamus waist" in a pneumoencephalogram. The floor of the central part of the lateral ventricle is formed medially by the "lamina affixa" and laterally by the body of the caudate nucleus. The roof consists of the corpus callosum. The choroid plexus extends through the interventricular foramen medially into the central part of the lateral ventricle. The central part of the lateral ventricle reaches the splenium of the corpus callosum, where it bifurcates into the occipital and temporal horns. Clinically, the junction of the occipital horn, the temporal horn, and the central part of the lateral ventricle is referred to as the collateral trigone or atrium (247). Anatomically, the latter (Fig. 13a.16) is a triangular area at the beginning of the temporal horn which lies in close topographic relationship to the deep collateral sulcus.

The occipital horn is covered by a radiation of the corpus callosum, the major forceps. An inward curvature on the medial wall of the occipital horn, the calcar avis, is caused by the calcarine sulcus.

The temporal horn deviates from the trigone in a small curve in a laterobasal direction. Located on its roof is the tail of the caudate nucleus. The amygdaloid body (amygdala) is found at the tip of the temporal horn (Figs. 9b.12 and 10b.21). The choroid plexus becomes part of the temporal horn on the medial side and extends to the fimbria of hippocampus. Mediobasally, the temporal horn is bordered by the hippocampus (Fig. 10b.24) with its alveus protruding into the temporal horn (Fig. 10b.23).

3.3 Arteries of the Brain and their Vascular Territories

(Figs. 28, 29, 30a–e, 31a, b, 5a–18a)

By following the course of the cerebral arteries in angiograms and by taking into account the variations in the arteries themselves, it is possible to localize the superficial and deep portions of the brain. Computed tomography generally does not provide a sufficient visualization of the cerebral blood vessels. In most cases, a cerebral angiogram is necessary when specific information is required. This is especially true in instances of vascular diseases, differential diagnosis of tumors, and for planning surgical intervention. In some cases, angiocomputed tomography alone is sufficient. Changes in vascular diseases and damage to the brain from edema, infarct, bleeding, and hydrocephalus can be recognized in computed tomographic examinations. Therefore, a three-dimensional correlation of the topographical anatomy of the cerebral arteries gained from frontal and lateral angiographic projections with the corresponding CT findings, derived from axial sections, is often necessary. To assist in this task, we have included a comparison of the angiograms of the most common arterial variations with the corresponding axial sections of the brain.

Occlusions of both large and small arteries of the brain are not immediately visualized in CT scans. After a few hours or days they may be seen as hypodense regions found in the areas supplied by the affected artery. The range and extent of hypodensity, recognized as a correlate in cases of edema and infarct, depends not only on the size of the occluded vessel but also on the extent of collateral blood supply. Aneurysms, having a diameter of 5 to 10 mm, may be detectable in CT scans (199). However, a contrast medium is usually necessary for their detection. Constantly reproducible evidence of an angioma is not provided by computed tomography.

Over the past few decades, a number of thorough studies has been completed to study the variability of the arteries of the brain (128, 143, 167, 168, 257, 259, 296, 310). Clinicians, however, have only partially adopted the international anatomical nomenclature and, as a result, synonyms are often used in publications. For this reason, in addition to the international anatomical nomenclature, synonyms are included in parentheses in this text.

Many of the anatomical names for the arteries of the brain are more than 100 years old. In many instances, a single conspicuous topographical feature was chosen as the basis for these names (11). "Cerebellar" arteries, which branch on the cerebellum, for example, send important circumferential branches to parts of the medulla oblongata, pons, and midbrain. As a result, proximal occlusions of a cerebellar artery may lead to dysfunctions in these four divisions of the brain. If we were to apply the mathematical set theory, names given to arteries of the brain frequently indicate only a subset of the set of regions supplied by a blood vessel.

The vertebral artery (Fig. 28) emerges from the atlas through the transverse foramen and runs initially in a dorsal direction before turning into the groove for the vertebral artery of the atlas (Fig. 5a.19). In this way, a "reserve loop" of the artery is formed, allowing for free movement of the head (35). This portion of the vertebral artery can be seen in the lateral view of an angiogram as V3 segment.

The vertebral artery extends diagonally from its groove through the atlantooccipital membrane, the dura mater, and the arachnoid. At this point the atlantooccipital sinus is attached to the ampulloglomerular organ, most likely a receptor apparatus for vascular reflexes. The vertebral artery continues in an arch and finally reaches the medulla oblongata (Fig. 6a.15). The intracranial portion of the artery is

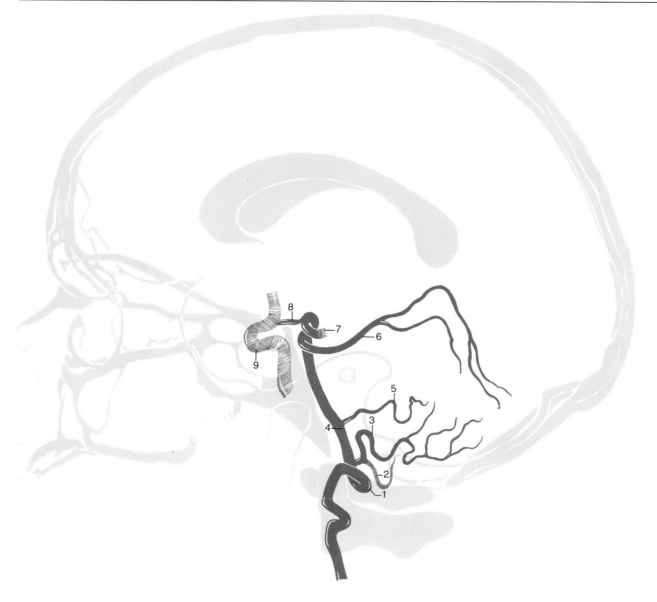

1 Vertebral artery
2 Variation of origin of posterior inferior cerebellar artery (PICA)
3 Posterior inferior cerebellar artery (PICA)
4 Basilar artery
5 Anterior inferior cerebellar artery (AICA)
6 Superior cerebellar artery
7 Posterior cerebral artery
8 Posterior communicating artery
9 Internal carotid artery

Fig. 28 Lateral view of the infratentorial arterial system with its connection to the internal carotid artery. According to (128).

referred to as V4 segment. The junction of the left and right vertebral arteries, forming the basilar artery, is located at the caudal edge of the pons in two-thirds of cases. In the remaining third, this junction is found on the rostral portion of the medulla oblongata. In the V4 segment either the right or the left vertebral artery may be somewhat wider or takes the form of a loop.

Angiographic examinations of the vertebral artery can demonstrate branches, namely the anterior spinal artery and the posterior inferior cerebellar artery. The anterior spinal artery branches off the vertebral artery just before the junction with the basilar artery and runs in a mediocaudal direction. In 77% of cases, the right and left arteries form an unpaired medial located anterior spinal artery approximately 2 cm from their origin (168). In 20% of cases, the anterior spinal artery is unilaterally absent and in about 13%, the contralateral branches do not join. Paramedian branches arise from the anterior spinal artery and extend towards the medulla oblongata.

The posterior inferior cerebellar artery (Fig. 6a.18), also referred to as PICA, generally arises intracranially from the vertebral artery, but in 18% of cases it arises extracranially caudal to the foramen magnum. In about 10% of all patients examined, the posterior inferior cerebellar artery arises not from the vertebral artery but from the basilar artery. The PICA is unilaterally absent in 10% of cases. A bilateral absence is recorded in only 2% of cases (168). This cerebellar artery takes a highly variable route along the lateral edge of the medulla oblongata (128, 168). It sends fine branches into the lateral segment of the medulla oblongata, where the nucleus ambiguus and other structures, such as the central sympathetic pathway, the spinal tract of the trigeminal nerve, and the spinothalamic tract are located. The posterior inferior cerebellar artery continues and occasionally forms loops on or around the tonsil of cerebellum. In 18% of cases, the PICA lies caudal to the foramen magnum (128). Therefore, a low caudal localization of these PICA loops does not indicate a brain edema complicated by a downward shift of the tonsils of cerebellum. One branch of this cerebellar artery extends into the choroid plexus of the fourth ventricle. The last portion of the posterior inferior cerebellar artery is located on the caudal surface of the cerebellum and branches into two directions: One branch supplies the caudal surface of the vermis and the other the caudal surface of the cerebellar hemisphere including a small part of the dentate nucleus.

The basilar artery is formed by the junction of the vertebral arteries. Located in the basilar sulcus of the pons, the basilar artery runs cranially through the pontine cistern and into the interpeduncular cistern (Figs. 7a.11, 8a.12, 9a.14). It is 15 to 40 mm long, on the average 32 mm. The cranial end of the basilar artery lies in 51% of cases at the level of the dorsum sellae, in 30% it is above it and in 19% below it (128). The artery forms a right or left concave arch in 10% of cases. This arch is usually combined with a thicker contralateral vertebral artery and is assumed, therefore, to be the result of existing hemodynamic factors (109). This curved course is not to be confused with a pathological displacement due to intracranial tumors.

Branches of the basilar artery are:

1. Pontine arteries (these fine branches are not cut in our sections, and hence are not included in the illustrations)
2. Anterior inferior cerebellar artery (Figs. 7a.15 and 8a.18)
3. Superior cerebellar artery (Fig. 9a.16)
4. Posterior cerebral artery (Fig. 9a.13).

The pontine arteries, in most cases about eight, arise almost at right angles from the basilar artery. Their medial branches supply the paramedian sector of the pons and the midbrain. The short circumferential branches partially supply the lateral sector of the pons. The pontine arteries are not generally seen in angiograms.

The anterior inferior cerebellar artery (AICA) originates in 52% of cases from the lower third of the basilar artery. In 46% of cases it arises from the middle third and in 2% from the upper third of the basilar artery. Exceptionally, the AICA arises from the vertebral artery. In 10% of cases there is a duplication of the AICA; in approximately 1% of cases it is unilaterally absent, only rarely it is bilaterally absent. The first part of the AICA usually extends laterocaudally over the pons and gives off a few fine branches. It then continues as a loop, from which in approximately 70% of cases the labyrinthine artery arises. In the remaining instances, the labyrinthine artery emerges directly from the basilar artery. The anterior inferior cerebellar artery either crosses the flocculus or encircles and supplies it with fine branches. From this floccular portion of the artery, additional fine branches extend into the pons and the medulla oblongata. The hemispheric branches of the anterior inferior cerebellar artery supply the caudal surface of the cerebellum as well as the choroid plexus of the fourth ventricle.

The superior cerebellar artery is the most form-constant cerebellar artery. It arises from the basilar artery just before its terminal bifurcation. In 4% of cases, this cerebellar artery arises from the posterior cerebral artery (167). In about 10%, the superior cerebellar artery is duplicated on both sides. The superior cerebellar artery gives off fine branches to parts of the pons, the superior cerebellar peduncle, and the tectal lamina (quadrigeminal plate). Thicker

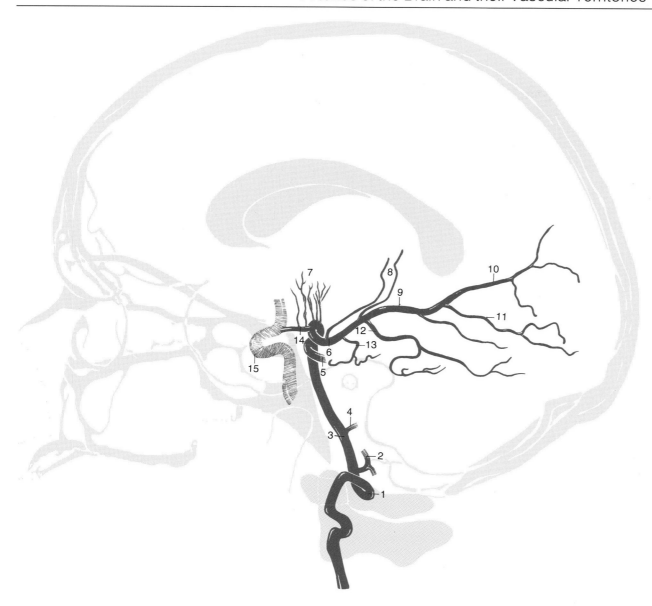

Fig. 29 Lateral view of the posterior cerebral artery. According to (128).

branches reach the cranial surface of the cerebellum. The cerebellar arteries are commonly joined through anastomoses.

In the case of an aplasia of a cerebellar artery, the group of cerebellar arteries has the ability of partial or complete compensation. With an aplasia of the PICA, for instance, the anterior inferior cerebellar artery and the superior cerebellar artery take over the blood supply to the caudal surface of the cerebellum. In 60% of cases, one posterior inferior cerebellar artery can independently supply the caudal surface of the cerebellum. The PICA is assisted in 26% of cases by the anterior inferior cerebellar artery and in 3% by the superior cerebellar artery. The cranial surface, on the other hand, is supplied in 67% of cases by the superior cerebellar artery. The anterior

inferior cerebellar artery and the PICA assist the superior cerebellar artery (168).

The posterior cerebral arteries (Figs. 29 and 9a.13) arise, in 90% of cases, as the terminal bifurcation of the basilar artery and reach into the interpeduncular cistern between the cerebral peduncles and the clivus. In the other 10% a fetal type is present, in which the posterior cerebral artery forms an extension of the posterior communicating artery. In this instance, the posterior cerebral artery is, in fact, a branch of the internal carotid artery.

The portion of the posterior cerebral artery between the basilar and the posterior communicating artery is referred to as the precommunicating portion of the posterior cerebral artery. It ranges from 3 to 9 mm in length, averaging 6 mm. The midbrain and diencephalon are partially supplied by small penetrating branches of the precommunicating portion. These thin arterial branches are seldom visible in angiograms (167).

The postcommunicating portion of the posterior cerebral artery arches around the midbrain and lies in the ambient cistern. The medial and lateral posterior choroid arteries arise at the beginning of the postcommunical part of the posterior cerebral artery (Fig. 10a.14). They run between the tectal lamina (quadrigeminal plate) and the parahippocampal gyrus and supply the choroid plexus of the third and lateral ventricles. In addition, thin branches run to the tectum (quadrigeminal plate), pineal gland, and to further portions of the diencephalon. Several branches reach the lateral and medial geniculate bodies and the dorsal side of the thalamus. These diencephalic arteries are also named penetrating branches (36, 110).

Between one and four hemispheric branches of the posterior cerebral artery supply the parahippocampal gyrus, the hippocampal formation, and parts of the splenium of the corpus callosum. In cerebral edema the tentorium of cerebellum may strangulate branches of the parahippocampal arteries because of transtentorial herniation. As a result, one sector of the hippocampal formation usually degenerates. This sector, the sector of Sommer, corresponds to the h1 field (180, 305). Additional hemispheric branches of the parahippocampal arteries run towards the caudal side of the temporal lobe. Underneath the posterior nucleus of the thalamus (otherwise known as the pulvinar thalami) and above the tentorium of cerebellum, the posterior cerebral artery divides into two hemispheric branches: the medial occipital artery (Figs. 10a.12, 11a.15, 12a.21) and the lateral occipital artery (occipitotemporal artery (128)) (Figs. 10a.13 and 11a.18). The division of the posterior cerebral artery into two approximately equally sized main branches generally takes place at the most lateral point of the cerebral peduncles. This division into a medial occipital artery and a lateral occipital artery is usually a bifurcation, seldom a trifurcation, and only exceptionally a quadrifurcation (167).

The lateral occipital artery reaches over the dorsal section of the parahippocampal gyrus supplying the caudal surface of the occipital lobe. The medial occipital artery runs beneath the splenium of the corpus callosum and crosses the isthmus of the cingulate gyrus. The artery divides into its terminal branches, namely the parieto-occipital and calcarine arteries. The parieto-occipital artery (Figs. 13a.21, 14a.16, 15a.15) runs, for the most part, in the sulcus of the same name and supplies the cuneus and precuneus. The calcarine artery (Figs. 12a.22 and 13a.23) lies on or in the calcarine sulcus. It arises only occasionally from the lateral occipital artery. The visual cortex is completely supplied by the cal-

carine artery in only 25% of all cases (281). In the remainder, the visual cortex is partially supplied by neighboring arteries. Vascular occlusions of the calcarine artery can give rise to a homonymous hemianopsia. The macula can be spared, if a neighboring artery sufficiently supplies the portion of the striate area that lies at the superior margin and has a point-to-point connection with the macula lutea.

The internal carotid artery (Figs. 30, 5a.11, 6a.12, 7a.9) enters the external skull base through the carotid canal in the petrosal portion of the temporal bone. The artery runs vertically at first, later it bends sharply in an anteromedial direction. It ascends a short distance almost in a vertical direction (C5 segment) through the cavernous sinus (Figs. 8a.10 and 8a.9). In the next section of its path, the internal carotid artery lies lateral to the pituitary fossa (C4 segment). The internal carotid artery curves backwards below the anterior clinoid process. The frontally directed convex arch forms the carotid genu (C3 segment, carotid knee). In recent publications the intracavernous section of the internal carotid artery is referred to as the juxtasellar segment (128). Passing through the dura mater and the arachnoid (C2 segment), the internal carotid artery enters the subarachnoid space in a dorsal direction. This subarachnoid part of the artery averages 13 mm in length, ranging from 8 to 18 mm (134). The next section reaches the point of its terminal bifurcation (C1 segment) into the anterior cerebral artery (Fig. 9a.10) and the middle cerebral artery (Fig. 9a.11). Direct branches of the internal carotid artery supply the optic chiasm, the pituitary stalk, the anterior lobe of the pituitary gland, as well as small portions of the hypothalamus, the genu of the internal capsule, and occasionally the globus pallidus and anterior portions of the thalamus (168).

The posterior communicating artery (Fig. 9a.12) arises from the internal carotid artery in the region between the sella turcica and the tuber cinereum of the diencephalon. It runs occipitally along the upper edge of the tentorium. In one out of a hundred cases, the posterior communicating artery is absent. In 10% of cases a fetal type is present in which the posterior communicating artery has such a large lumen that the posterior cerebral artery receives the principal portion of its blood from the internal carotid artery through the posterior communicating artery (167). Branches of the posterior communicating artery supply the optic chiasm, portions of the optic tract, the mamillary body, the tuber cinereum, additional portions of the hypothalamus, the thalamus between the interthalamic adhesion (intermediate mass) and the interventricular foramen (Monro), the cerebral peduncles, and the tail of the caudate nucleus.

The anterior choroid artery almost always arises from the internal carotid artery distal to the posterior communicating artery and about 3 mm proximal to the bifurcation of the internal carotid artery (167). Exceptionally, the anterior choroid artery arises from the posterior communicating artery. Approximately 25 mm long, the anterior choroid artery extends between the optic tract and the parahippocampal gyrus, enters the interpeduncular cistern and runs through the ambient cistern to the top of the temporal horn of the lateral ventricle into the choroid plexus. Fine branches of the anterior choroid artery reach the uncus of the parahippocampal gyrus, the amygdaloid body, the internal portion of the globus pallidus, as well as the posterior limb of the internal capsule, in which the corticonuclear and corticospinal tracts are located.

The anterior cerebral artery (Figs. 30, 9a.10, 10a.6, 11a.5, 12a.7) arises with the middle cerebral artery from the terminal bifurcation of the internal carotid artery. This bifurcation lies in the cleft between the optic chiasm and the anterior pole of the temporal lobe in the region of the anterior clinoid process. Aplasia of the anterior cerebral artery is observed in less than 1% of cases (167). The anterior cerebral artery curves anteromedially, and thereafter it is located above the optic nerve. The initial, precommunicating portion (A1 segment) of the anterior cerebral artery averages 14 mm in length (167) and reaches the anterior communicating artery. The second section, the postcommunicating portion (A2 segment), begins distal to its connection with the anterior communicating artery.

Several short central (medial lenticulostriate (15)) arteries arise from the precommunicating portion of the anterior cerebral artery and penetrate the anterior perforated substance. The long central artery (Heubner's artery) arises predominantly from the postcommunicating portion. In only 10% of cases it arises from the precommunicating portion (168). These central or penetrating branches supply deep structures of the forebrain: lamina terminalis, anterior commissure, anterior nuclei of the hypothalamus, anterior limb of the internal capsule, anterior portion of the globus pallidus, and anteroinferior part of the head of the caudate nucleus.

Hemispheric branches from the postcommunicating portion of the anterior cerebral artery extend into the cerebral cortex and the adjacent white matter. The medial frontobasal artery (Figs. 9a.5 and 30.4) arises near the subcallosal area and supplies the medial portion of the orbital forebrain. The frontopolar artery (Fig. 10a.3) extends diagonally in a rostral direction toward the frontal pole. This artery is used as a point of reference in the interpretation of angiograms (257). The horizontally running terminal part of the anterior cerebral artery is known as the pericallosal artery (Figs. 13a.8 and 14a.10) (246).

Further branching of the anterior cerebral artery generally takes one of the two forms (128):

1. A principal branch of the anterior cerebral artery, the callosomarginal artery (Figs. 12a.5, 13a.6, 14a.7, 15a.7), lies in the cingulate sulcus and gives off branches (Fig. 30a).
2. The branches may arise directly from the anterior cerebral artery or from the pericallosal artery (Fig. 30b).

The hemispheric branches of the anterior cerebral artery supply the medial surface of the frontal and parietal lobes almost as far as the parieto-occipital sulcus. The additional region supplied by the anterior cerebral artery is a longitudinal, 2 to 3 cm wide territory overlapping the superior margin of the hemisphere including the superior frontal gyrus, the rostral portion of the middle frontal gyrus, the portions of the pre- and postcentral gyri near the superior margin, and a part of the superior parietal lobule. Additionally, the corpus callosum, with the exception of the splenium, is supplied by the anterior cerebral artery.

The anterior communicating artery (Fig. 9a.9) forms a connection, about 3 mm in length, between the right and left anterior cerebral arteries. It is located above the optic chiasm at the level of the anterior clinoid process. Fine branches supply the optic chiasm, the infundibulum, and the preoptic regions of the hypothalamus.

The middle cerebral artery (Figs. 31 and 9a.11) is a continuation of the internal carotid artery running from its medial point of origin deep into the cistern of the lateral (Sylvian) fissure. The initial or sphenoid portion (M1 segment) of the middle cerebral artery is located just below the anterior perforated substance. Here 3 to 13 thin arteries, the anterolateral central (lateral lenticulostriate (16)) arteries, branch off mainly to supply deeper telencephalic and diencephalic structures: the genu and posterior limb of the internal capsule, the majority of the putamen and caudate nucleus, and part of the globus pallidus.

Prior to its division into two or more branches, the middle cerebral artery stretches on the average 16 mm (5 to 24 mm). Aplasia of the middle cerebral artery is reported rarely and is seen only in about 0.3% of the cases examined (167). In the region between the anterior perforated substance and the insula, the middle cerebral artery divides into its hemispheric branches as a bifurcation in 20% of cases (Fig. 31a), as a trifurcation in about 50% (Fig. 31b); only seldom does it form a quadrifurcation or quintafurcation (167). The insular arteries (Figs. 10a.7, 11a.6, 12a.9, 13a.10) ascend dorsally in an oblique manner and lie on the insula (M2 segment). They run around the frontal, parietal, and temporal opercula. During evolution the neocortex pushed the opercula over the insula together with these arteries (285, 287). The arteries enclose the

1 Internal carotid artery
2 Branches of middle
  cerebral artery
3 Anterior cerebral artery
4 Medial frontobasal artery
5 Callosomarginal artery
6 Frontopolar artery
7 Anteromedial (anterior
  internal (128)) frontal
  artery
8 Mediomedial (middle internal (128)) frontal artery
9 Pericallosal artery
10 Posteromedial (posterior
   internal (128)) frontal
   artery
11 Paracentral artery
12 Superior precuneal
   (superior internal
   parietal (128)) artery
13 Inferior precuneal (inferior
   internal parietal (128))
   artery

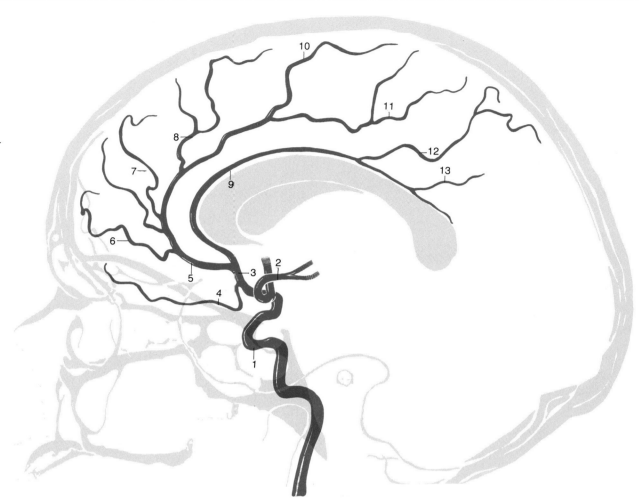

Fig. 30a and **b**   Lateral view of two main variations of the anterior cerebral artery: a) secondary branches originate from the callosomarginal artery, a main branch of the anterior cerebral artery; b) secondary branches arise directly from the anterior cerebral artery. According to (128).

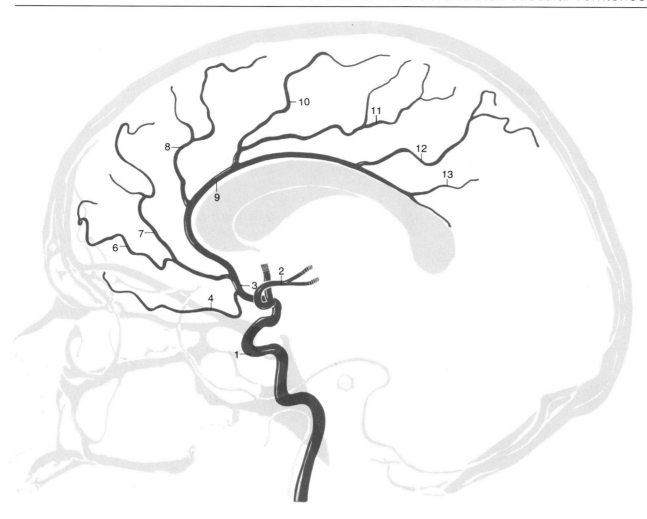

opercula of the insula (M3 segment) and assume the shape of a candelabra. The concave portion of the curve in the ascending arteries is directed upward. Likewise, in descending arteries of the temporal operculum the concave portion of the candelabra is directed downward. The terminal segments of the insular arteries lie on the surface of the cerebrum (M4 and M5 segments). The hemispheric branches are named according to the region that they supply peripherally.

The lateral frontobasal artery (Fig. 31.4) supplies the inferior frontal gyrus and partially the orbital gyri. The prefrontal artery (Figs. 13a.5, 14a.5, 15a.5) lies on the triangular part of the operculum and branches on the external surface of the frontal lobe. The artery to the precentral sulcus (Prerolandic artery) (Figs. 12a.8, 13a.9, 14a.8, 15a.8) lies to some extent in the precentral sulcus and supplies the middle frontal gyrus and the basilar part of the precentral gyrus. The artery to the central sulcus (Rolandic artery) (Figs. 13a.14, 14a.9, 15a.9) assists in supplying the precentral and postcentral gyri as well as the adjacent areas. The anterior and posterior parietal arteries supply the anterior and posterior parts of the parietal lobe. The angular artery (Figs. 13a.19, 14a.15, 15a.14) runs partially in the superior temporal sulcus in the direction of the angular gyrus and can be seen as the terminal branch of the middle cerebral artery. There are three temporal arteries that descend along the surface of the temporal lobe. The temporo-occipital artery runs on the superior temporal gyrus to the occipital lobe.

In all but 4% of cases, the circle of Willis forms a vascular ring joining the blood flow systems of basilar and internal carotid arteries. The circle can act as an adaptive distributor during variations in the blood supply of one of the arteries (142). In about 2% of cases, the left or right posterior communicating artery is absent (168). Hemodynamically speaking, connections between the large cerebral arteries are not sufficient in about 50% of cases (4). The preferred localization of arteriosclerosis in the cerebral arterial circle can further impair its compensational functions (306). In adults a complete ligation of one internal carotid artery generally results in neurologic deficits.

1 Internal carotid artery
2 Middle cerebral artery
3 Anterior cerebral artery
4 Lateral frontobasal artery
5 Insular arteries
6 Prefrontal arteries
7 Artery to precentral sulcus
   (Prerolandic artery (128))
8 Artery to central sulcus
   (Rolandic artery (128))
9 Anterior parietal artery
10 Posterior parietal artery
11 Angular artery
12 Temporo-occipital artery
   (128)
13 Posterior temporal artery
14 Middle temporal artery
15 Anterior temporal artery
16 Temporal polar artery
   (128)

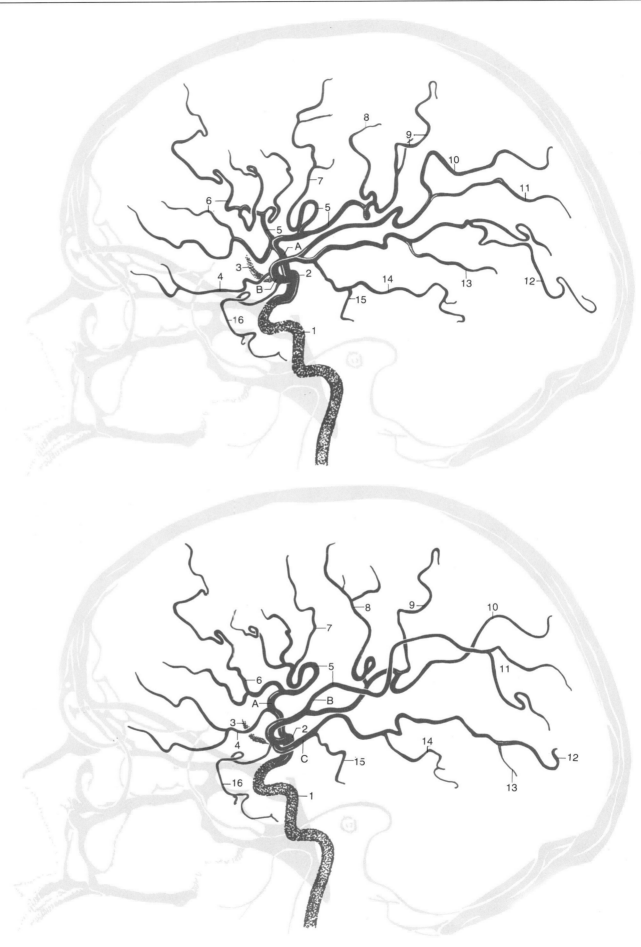

Fig. 31a and **b**   Lateral view of two variations of the middle cerebral artery: a) with a bifurcation A, B; b) with a trifurcation A, B, C. According to (128).

Most cerebral arteries have arterial interconnections (anastomoses) which can partially supply neighboring brain areas. Hemodynamically the most important anastomosis is the circle of Willis. The protective importance of the circle of Willis is illustrated by the fact that a congenitally incomplete circle of Willis is significantly more common among patients who have had strokes. Furthermore, leptomeningeal anastomoses between the three main cerebral arteries and the three cerebellar arteries are of functional importance. Across the midline a compensational supply is possible through the pericallosal artery or the callosomarginal artery. Arterial anastomoses can also develop between the anterior choroid artery and the posterior choroid artery.

Many other areas of anastomotic supply are known (128). But if an occlusion of a large cerebral vessel occurs suddenly, generally the collaterals do not suffice to supply that vascular territory. A severe hypoperfusion leads to a softening of brain tissue (ischemic stroke). The clinical symptoms of an arterial occlusion depend on the neurofunctional systems which are affected. The knowledge of the topography of the arterial territories, as well as of the neurofunctional systems is necessary in neurological medicine.

The arterial supply of the brain stem is divided into medial (also called paramedian, due to its localization) and lateral territories. In the medulla oblongata the medial territory is supplied by the anterior spinal arteries and through direct branches of the vertebral arteries. This territory holds the pyramidal tract and the hypoglossal nucleus. A unilateral lesion of the medial territory causes a pyramidal contralateral hemiparesis and an ipsilateral nuclear/infranuclear hypoglossal paralysis. The pyramidal tract crosses caudally to this lesion, whereas the motoneurons of the hypoglossal nerve reach the muscles of the tongue on the same side. The syndrome of a "crossed" paralyses makes a neuroanatomical localization possible.

The lateral territory of the medulla oblongata is supplied by fine branches of the cerebellar arteries and includes the following neurofunctional systems: the spinal nucleus of the trigeminal nerve, the spinothalamic tract, the vestibular nuclei, and emerging fibers of the glossopharyngeal and vagus nerves. The syndrome of the "crossed" disorders of pain and temperature sensation of the face, limbs, and trunk has already been mentioned as Wallenberg's syndrome. Here the lesion of the trigeminal system has ipsilateral effects and that of the spinothalamic tract contralateral effects, because the unilateral lesion in the medulla oblongata is located before the crossing of the trigeminal system and after the crossing of the spinothalamic tract. Infarction in the vestibular system leads to vertigo, vomiting, and nausea. A lesion of the ninth and tenth cranial nerves may present with dysphagia and hoarseness (paralysis of pharyngeal and laryngeal muscles).

In the pons we can differentiate as well a medial territory, supplied by the pontine arteries (paramedian branches of the basilar artery), and a lateral territory, supplied by the small branches of the anterior inferior cerebellar artery and the superior cerebellar artery.

In the forebrain a similar but more complicated order of arterial territories exists. From the circle of Willis numerous small arteries branch off into the paramedian territory of the forebrain. Small penetrating branches arise from the proximal portions of the anterior, middle, and posterior cerebral arteries. These end-arteries lack anastomotic interconnections, and occlusion of individual vessels causes small infarcts.

The penetrating branches of the anterior cerebral artery include Heubner's artery and anteromedial central (medial lenticulostriate (15)) arteries. They supply the anteroinferior part of caudate nucleus and putamen and the anteroinferior part of the internal capsule (15) (Fig. 31e).

The penetrating branches of the middle cerebral artery supply the substantia innominata, lateral part of the anterior commissure, most of the putamen, and lateral portion of the globus pallidus, superior half of the internal capsule and adjacent corona radiata, body and head (except the anteroinferior part) of caudate nucleus (16) (Fig. 31e).

The penetrating branches of the posterior cerebral artery and circle of Willis supply the thalamus, metathalamus, hypothalamus and subthalamic nucleus. Further, penetrating branches of the posterior cerebral artery reach parts of the mesencephalon (110) (Fig. 31e).

Occlusion of a penetrating artery can produce a well-circumscribed infarct. If only the pyramidal tract is affected, a contralateral hemiplegia without sensory disturbances will develop. Infarcts in the ventral posterior nucleus of the thalamus produce "pure hemisensory loss".

The vascular territories of the hemispheric branches of the anterior, middle, and posterior cerebral arteries are demonstrated in Figures 31c and d. The anterior cerebral artery supplies the anterior three-quarters of the medial surface of the cerebral hemisphere up to the level of the parieto-occipital sulcus. Furthermore, it supplies the anterior four-fifths of the corpus callosum with the exception of the splenium. Additional small branches supply a 2 to 3 cm wide strip along the convexity of the hemisphere along the superior margin. This area includes the superior frontal gyrus, the parts of the pre- and postcentral gyri close to the superior margin, as well as the upper parietal gyri. These vascular territories of the cortex and adjacent white matter contain the following neurofunctional systems: primary motor

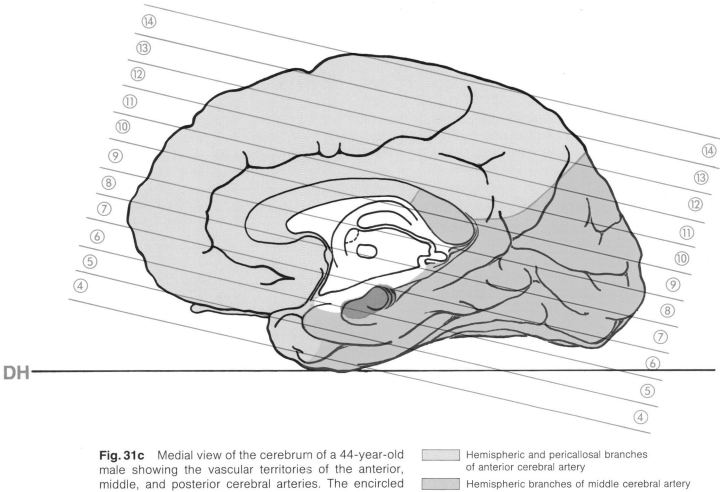

Fig. 31c Medial view of the cerebrum of a 44-year-old male showing the vascular territories of the anterior, middle, and posterior cerebral arteries. The encircled number indicates the number of the slice.
DH = Reid's base line = "Deutsche Horizontale". According to (15, 16, 51, 110).

Hemispheric and pericallosal branches of anterior cerebral artery

Hemispheric branches of middle cerebral artery

Hemispheric and callosal branches of posterior cerebral artery

Anterior choroid artery

and sensory area of the contralateral leg. Occlusions of the hemispheric branches of the anterior cerebral artery cause a contralateral weakness and sensory loss of the leg. If the patient's language areas are located in the left hemisphere and an anterior cerebral artery is occluded, verbal commands can no longer be conducted to the still functioning primary motor cortex of the right hemisphere, because their connection in the corpus callosum is severed (disconnection syndrome).

The hemispheric branches of the middle cerebral artery supply the insula, the frontal, parietal, and temporal opercula and an oval territory around the lateral sulcus (Fig. 31d). This territory includes the primary motor and sensory areas of the trunk, arm, and head. Furthermore, the middle cerebral artery supplies the white matter beneath the frontal, parietal, and temporal cortical areas. The upper part of the optic radiation (geniculocalcarine tract) is located in the parietal white matter and the lower part in the temporal white matter. The frontal oper-

culum holds Broca's area. The superior temporal gyrus in the temporal operculum includes Wernicke's area.

Infarction in the territory of the middle cerebral artery causes contralateral weakness and sensory loss of the trunk, arm, and head, as well as contralateral inferior quadrantanopsia (interruption of the parietal optic radiation) or contralateral superior quadrantanopsia (interruption of the temporal optic radiation). If the language areas in the dominant hemisphere are affected, a motor language disorder (Broca's aphasia) or a sensory language disorder (Wernicke's aphasia) may result. When opercular damage is widespread, there results a severe language disturbance of a mixed type (global aphasia (36)).

The hemispheric branches of the posterior cerebral artery supply the inferior temporal lobe and large parts of the occipital lobe on its medial surface, especially the visual cortex (Fig. 31c). At the convexity of the hemispheres a small strip of the occipital

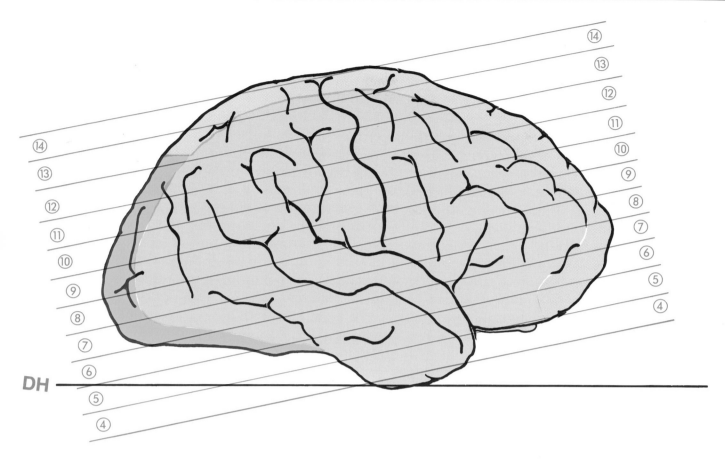

Fig. 31d   Lateral view of the cerebrum of a 44-year-old male showing the vascular territories of the anterior, middle, and posterior cerebral arteries. The encircled number indicates the number of the slice.
DH = Reid's base line = "Deutsche Horizontale"
According to (15, 16, 51, 110).

Hemispheric branches of anterior cerebral artery
Hemispheric branches of middle cerebral artery
Hemispheric branches of posterior cerebral artery

and temporal lobes are supplied by them as well (Fig. 31d). An occlusion of the posterior cerebral artery causes a contralateral homonymous hemianopsia. The posterior cerebral artery also supplies the splenium of the corpus callosum. A lesion of the splenium leads to the disconnection of the primary visual cortex of the nondominant hemisphere from the language areas of the dominant hemisphere. These patients may develop problems reading (alexia due to disconnection).

In Figures 31c–e the vascular territories of cerebral arteries are demonstrated according to references (15, 16, 36, 51, 110, 128, 168, 257, 296, 310). They are simplified and an average size was chosen. Individual variations have to be taken into account. The extent of an infarct depends on the respective collateral supply.

Hemispheric and pericallosal branches of anterior cerebral artery

Hemispheric branches of middle cerebral artery

Hemispheric branches of posterior cerebral artery

Penetrating branches of anterior cerebral artery

Penetrating branches of middle cerebral artery

Penetrating branches of posterior cerebral artery and posterior communicating artery

Anterior choroid artery

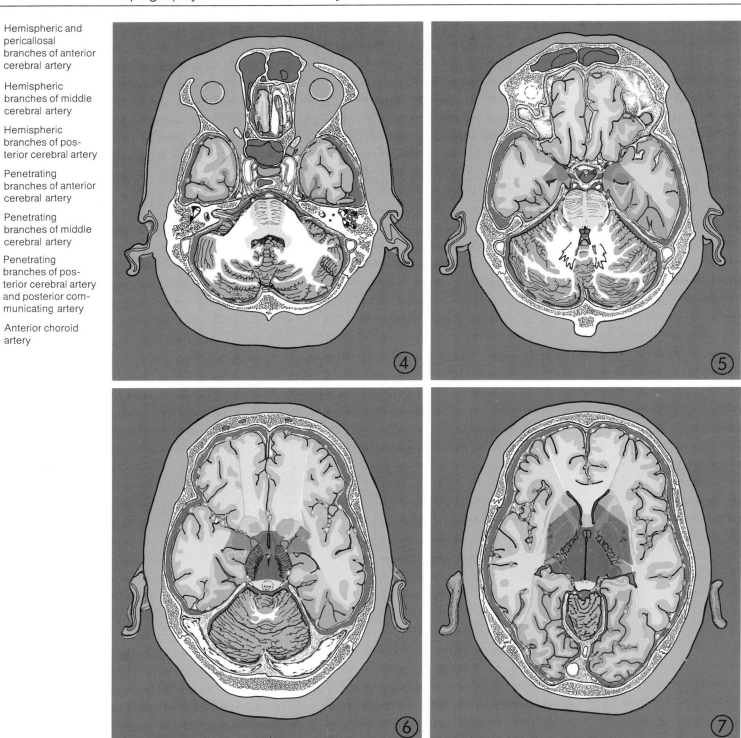

Fig. 31e Serial illustrations showing the vascular territories of the anterior, middle, and posterior cerebral arteries and the anterior choroid artery. The encircled number indicates the number of the slice. According to (15, 16, 51, 110).

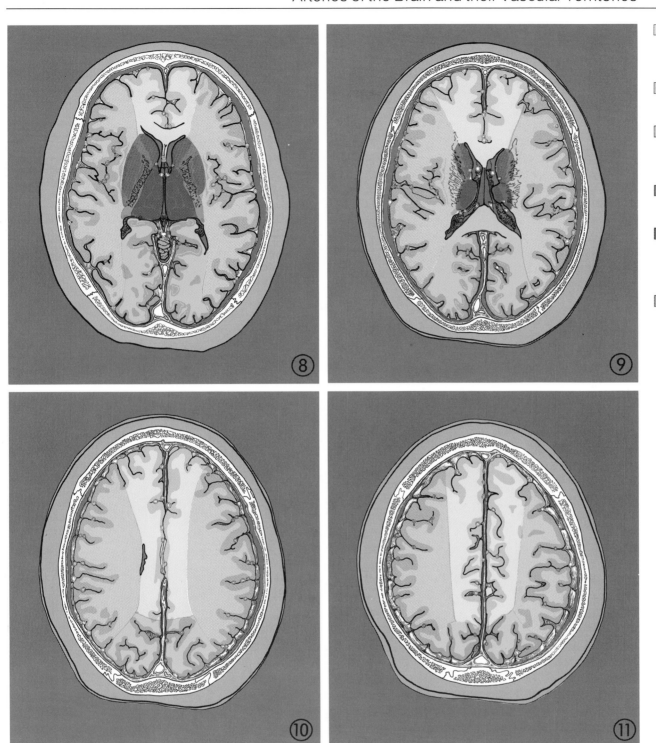

Hemispheric and pericallosal branches of anterior cerebral artery

Hemispheric branches of middle cerebral artery

Hemispheric and callosal branches of posterior cerebral artery

Penetrating branches of middle cerebral artery

Penetrating branches of posterior cerebral artery and posterior communicating artery

Anterior choroid artery

Hemispheric
branches of anterior
cerebral artery

Hemispheric
branches of middle
cerebral artery

Hemispheric
branches of pos-
terior cerebral artery

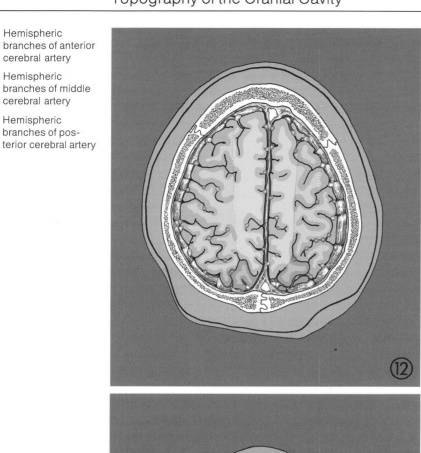

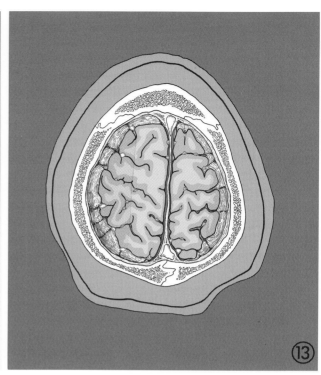

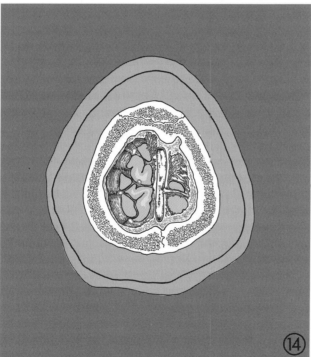

Fig. 31e Serial illustrations showing the vascular territories of the anterior, middle, and posterior cerebral arteries and the anterior choroid artery. The encircled number indicates the number of the slice. According to (15, 16, 51, 110).

3.4 Veins of the Brain

(Figs. 32, 33, 5a–18a)

In the human body numerous veins run along common vascular routes parallel to their corresponding arteries. The veins of the brain, however, run spatially independent of the arteries of the brain. In addition, these veins also show a greater variability than the arteries. Nevertheless, the topography of veins can be described by a general scheme. The topography of the deep intracerebral veins, as shown in angiograms, is of particular diagnostic importance. In the venous phase of the angiogram, space occupying lesions can be recognized by the displacement of the deep cranial veins. The superficial arteries of the brain may appear normal in such angiographic images.

The veins and sinuses can be used to some extent as guideline structures in computed tomography (Chap. 2.5.5). Pathological changes or displacements are frequently discrete or not visible at all. Dislocations of the medial structures are often more clearly identified by changes of the ventricular system than by displacement of the veins.

The veins of the brain contain no valves and form a tubular network with many anastomoses. The principal venous drainage occurs via the venous sinuses through the internal jugular vein (Figs. 5a.13, 6a.13, 7a.17). The internal jugular vein leaves the skull through the jugular foramen (Figs. 7a.16 and 21.16). Other veins can take over the drainage of the internal jugular veins. The internal vertebral venous plexus can drain blood from a basilar venous plexus located on the clivus. The cavernous sinus may drain through the ophthalmic veins into the facial vein. Cerebral blood can, furthermore, be drained into the pterygoid plexus via the veins passing through the oval foramen, via veins located in the carotid canal (not indicated in Figure 32), and via emissary veins. The telencephalon and diencephalon are drained by two groups of veins:

1. Superficial veins drain blood mainly from the cortical areas.
2. Deep veins receive most of their blood from the white matter and the nuclear regions located there. In a few instances, these deep veins also drain the cortical regions. Blood from the branches of the deep veins is collected in a cascading manner in the great cerebral vein (Galen) (Figs. 12a.19 and 13a.20). This large vein usually joins the inferior sagittal sinus (Fig. 32.11) at its junction with the straight sinus (Fig. 32.13) (168).

The superficial cerebral veins include the superior cerebral veins (Figs. 12a.3, 13a.3, 14a.3, 15a.3, 16a.4), inferior cerebral veins, and superficial middle cerebral veins (Figs. 10a.5 and 11a.9). The superior cerebral veins, known simply as the superficial cerebral veins, ascend in an arch along the curvature of the cerebral hemisphere to join the superior sagittal sinus (Figs. 11a.2, 12a.2, 13a.2, 14a.2, 15a.2, 16a.2, 17a.2, 18a.5). The veins close to the sinus break through the arachnoid and fasten their adventitia to the tough connective tissue of the dura mater. These veins are referred to as "bridging veins" (Fig. 11a.3). They are subjected easily to mechanical injury and can be the source of a subdural hematoma (94, 156, 160).

The superficial cerebral veins are divided into prefrontal, frontal, parietal, and occipital branches. The inferior cerebral veins descend from the external surfaces of the frontal, temporal, and occipital lobes. The frontal veins generally flow into the superficial middle cerebral vein. The temporal and occipital veins flow directly into the transverse sinus (Fig. 10a.19) or indirectly via the posterior anastomotic veins. The superficial middle cerebral vein originates on the lateral wall of the cerebral hemisphere above the lateral sulcus. It may join the cavernous sinus (Fig. 8a.9), sphenoparietal sinus, the veins of the oval foramen, paracavernous sinus, superior petrosal sinus (Fig. 9a.19), or sigmoid sinus (Figs. 7a.19, 8a.20, 9a.20).

The great cerebral vein (Galen), which is approximately 1 cm long, collects the blood of the deep cerebral veins. It originates at the junction of both internal cerebral veins (Fig. 12a.12), curves around the posterior surface of the splenium of the corpus callosum, and usually terminates by draining into the region joining the inferior sagittal sinus and the straight sinus. At this point, the cerebral falx meets the ridge of the tentorium of the cerebellum.

The internal cerebral vein is the confluence of the anterior vein of the septum pellucidum (Fig. 12a.11), superior thalamostriate vein, also known as terminal vein (Fig. 13a.11), and the superior choroidal vein (Fig. 13a.12). The entry of the anterior vein of the septum pellucidum into the superior thalamostriate vein can be observed in lateral projections of the brain. This junction is referred to as the venous angle. It is usually located at the level of the interventricular foramen (Monro). Dislocation of the venous angle indicates an intracranial displacement especially in the median plane. The superior thalamostriate vein lies in about 50% of cases between the caudate nucleus and the thalamus. It may change its course in an occipital direction before it reaches the interventricular foramen. In this case, the confluence of the anterior vein of the septum pellucidum and the superior thalamostriate vein at the venous angle is located several millimeters occipital to the interventricular foramen (Monro) (168).

The internal cerebral vein runs dorsally inside the cistern of the transverse fissure (cistern of the velum interpositum) (168, 325) in a slightly wavelike man-

Superficial veins of cortical regions and their sinuses:
1 Superior (superficial) cerebral veins
2 Superior sagittal sinus
3 Superficial middle cerebral vein
4 Cavernous sinus
5 Inferior petrosal sinus

Deep veins of central and nuclear regions and their sinuses:
6 Anterior vein of septum pellucidum
7 Superior thalamostriate (terminal) vein
8 Venous angle
9 Internal cerebral vein
10 Great cerebral vein (Galen)
11 Inferior sagittal sinus
12 Basal vein (Rosenthal)
13 Straight sinus
14 Confluence of sinuses
15 Transverse sinus
16 Sigmoid sinus
17 Internal jugular vein

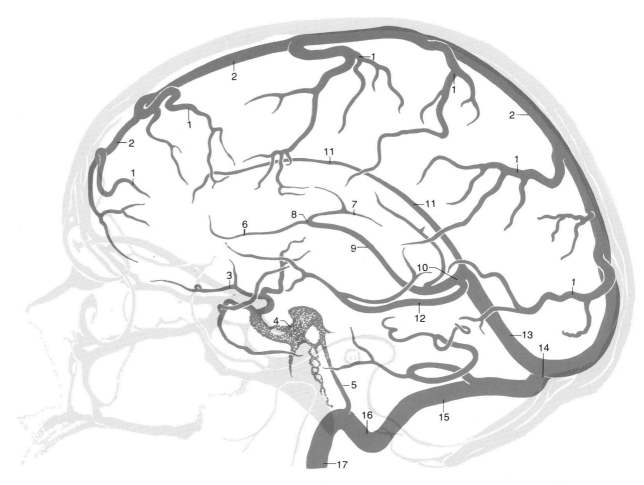

Fig. 32 Lateral view of the head illustrating the arrangement of veins and sinuses. The sequence of the numbers takes into account both the areas drained by the veins and the direction of blood flow. According to (128).

ner. Approximately 3.5 cm dorsal to the interventricular foramen, the right and left internal cerebral veins join to form the great cerebral vein (Galen). Dislocations of an internal cerebral vein visible in angiograms indicate a supratentorial displacement of a cerebral hemisphere.

The basal vein (Rosenthal) (Figs. 9a.15, 10a.15, 11a.19) is formed by various confluences: the anterior cerebral vein, the inferior central veins, and the deep cerebral vein of the anterior perforated substance. These veins receive blood from the basal and medial parts of the frontal lobe, the basal ganglia, and the insular regions. The basal vein runs occipitally along the optic tract between the cerebral peduncle and the diencephalon. The vein ascends dorsally around the cerebral peduncle in the ambient cistern.

In addition to the above mentioned drainage of the frontal and insular parts of the telencephalon, the initial basilar segment of the basal vein receives blood from the pole of the temporal lobe, hippocampus, as well as from portions of the midbrain and diencephalon. The second laterodorsal segment of the basal vein is located between the cerebral peduncle and its variable junction with either the internal cerebral vein, the great cerebral vein (Galen), or the straight sinus. The second segment receives venous blood from the cerebral peduncle, the tectum, the geniculate bodies, the body and splenium of the corpus callosum, the medial surface of the occipital lobe, and portions of the cerebellum.

The unpaired vessels, namely the great cerebral vein (Galen) and the straight sinus, collect blood from the paired internal cerebral veins and the basal veins. These veins drain the large regions of the white matter of the telencephalon, diencephalon, striatum,

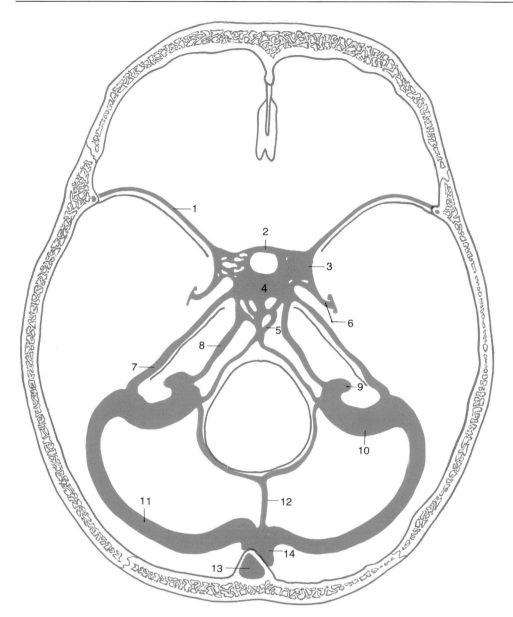

Fig. 33 Arrangement of the basal sinuses. According to (128).

midbrain, pons, cerebellum, and medial and basal regions of the frontal, temporal, and occipital surfaces of the telencephalon.

The straight sinus unites with the superior sagittal sinus at the confluence of sinuses (Fig. 11a.25) to form the transverse sinus. From there the venous blood flows via the sigmoid sinus into the internal jugular vein.

Blood generally drains from the midbrain through the great cerebral vein (Galen). Furthermore, small veins originating in the upper anterior portion of the cerebellum flow into the great cerebral vein. The large veins of the cerebellum run through the subarachnoid space independently of the arteries and join various blood vessels of the posterior cranial fossa.

The petrosal vein drains the lower anterior portions of the cerebellum and of the pons. This vein flows into the superior petrosal sinus. The remaining cerebellar veins drain into the straight sinus, the confluence of sinuses, and occasionally into the transverse sinus. Venous drainage of the pons and the medulla oblongata varies greatly, taking place through branches of the basal vein, the transverse sinus, the inferior and superior petrosal sinuses, the occipital sinus, or the internal vertebral venous plexus.

In isolated cases, a small hyperdense lesion in the CT scan will indicate a sinus thrombosis or a thrombotic occlusion of a large vein. On postinfusion scans the thrombus appears as a lucent, triangular-shaped defect in the superior sagittal sinus. As a rule, pathological density patterns due to reactive changes in the surrounding area are the only indication of a possible thrombophlebitis (199). Cerebral angiograms or digital intravenous subtraction angiography provide supporting evidence for such a diagnosis.

3.5 Cranial Nerves

The cranial nerves emerge from the base of the brain and pass through the subarachnoid space before penetrating the dura mater and leaving through the foramina in the skull base. The second cranial nerve is the only one retaining its sheath of dura mater outside the cranial cavity. Cranial nerves XII through VII leave via foramina in the posterior cranial fossa. Cranial nerves VI through II leave via foramina in the middle cranial fossa. The first cranial nerve passes through the cribriform plate, thus emerging from the anterior cranial fossa. The hypoglossal or twelfth cranial nerve (Fig. 6b.5) appears as 12 to 16 rootlets sprouting out of the medulla oblongata between the pyramid and olive. These rootlets join to form several bundles, which, as a rule, lie dorsal to the vertebral artery and extend as far as the hypoglossal canal of the occipital bone. The hypoglossal nerve innervates the muscles of the tongue.

The accessory or eleventh cranial nerve (Fig. 7b.10) has two roots: the spinal and the bulbar (cranial) roots. The fibers of the spinal root (Figs. 5b.4, 6b.6, 7b.11) arise from the C1 through C6 (maximal C7, minimal C3) segments of the spinal cord. They emerge from the lateral side of the spinal cord and extend cranially and pass through the foramen magnum to the posterior cranial fossa. The fibers of the cranial root arise as 3 to 6 rootlets on the lateral side of the medulla oblongata. Both roots join up with the ninth and tenth cranial nerves just proximal to the dural opening above the jugular foramen. These three nerves XI, X, and IX leave as a common trunk through the medial part of the jugular foramen. The spinal root of the accessory nerve innervates together with direct branches of the cervical plexus the ipsilateral sternocleidomastoid and trapezoid muscles. The cranial root assists in the motor innervation of the pharynx and partially innervates the muscles of the larynx.

The vagus or tenth cranial nerve (Fig. 7b.9) emerges from the lateral edge of the medulla oblongata by 10 to 18 fine rootlets. It stretches about 1.5 cm within a cistern to the dural opening above the jugular foramen (168). It conveys sensory information from a small area in the external acoustic (auditory) meatus and the sensory taste buds in the pharynx. It also carries visceral afferent information from the mucous membranes of the thoracic viscera and abdominal organs. The vagus nerve provides most of the motor innervation of the laryngeal muscles and partial innervation of the pharyngeal muscles. It is the parasympathetic nerve of the thoracic viscera, the upper abdominal organs, and intestinal tract up to the point of Cannon and Böhm.

The glossopharyngeal or ninth cranial nerve (Fig. 7b.9) has some morphological similarities with the vagus nerve. These similarities include a lateral exit from the medulla oblongata and a passage through the jugular foramen. Likewise, the glossopharyngeal nerve supplies the primary visceral regions including the mucosa of the palate and pharynx, the taste buds on the posterior third of the tongue, as well as the parasympathetic innervation of the parotid gland and a portion of the pharyngeal muscles.

The vestibulocochlear or eighth cranial nerve (Fig. 8b.15) (statoacoustic nerve) is a combination of two pathways: one serves the vestibular system, the other the auditory system. Following the direction of the afferent fibers, the nerve passes through the internal acoustic (auditory) meatus and enters the medulla oblongata at the lateral edge near the border with the pons. The intracisternal portion of the vestibulocochlear nerve is approximately 1.4 cm long (168).

The facial or seventh cranial nerve arises together with the intermediate nerve (Wrisberg) (Fig. 8b.14) from the lateral wall between pons and medulla oblongata. The intermediate nerve is an extremely thin bundle that runs in a caudal position parallel to the main part of the seventh cranial nerve. The seventh cranial nerve lies cranial to the vestibulocochlear nerve in the internal acoustic (auditory) meatus. The facial nerve measures approximately 1.6 cm from its origin to the internal acoustic meatus (168). The intermediate nerve contains sensory nerve fibers from the taste buds on the anterior two-thirds of the tongue and parasympathetic fibers for the lacrimal glands, the nasopharyngeal, sublingual, and submandibular glands. The facial nerve is principally motoric and innervates the muscles of facial expression, the stapedius muscle, and the posterior belly of the digastric muscle. In one out of three cases, the anterior inferior cerebellar artery forms a loop in the direct vicinity of the facial nerve. This vascular loop may lead to a compression of the facial nerve resulting in a hemifacial spasm (134, 234, 261).

The abducens nerve, trochlear nerve, and oculomotor nerve (cranial nerves VI, IV, and III, respectively) innervate the ocular muscles. The abducens nerve (Fig. 7b.5) arises from the basilar surface of the brain stem at the border between pons and medulla oblongata. It passes through the basilar cistern in front of the pons and enters the dura mater (Fig. 8b.11) at the clivus mediobasal to the tip of the petrous portion of the temporal bone. The intracisternal portion of the abducens nerve is 1.5 cm long (168). It continues through the venous basilar plexus and enters the lateral wall of the cavernous sinus. It then leaves the middle cranial fossa through the superior orbital fissure and innervates the lateral rectus muscle. A lesion of the abducens nerve leads to an ipsilateral strabismus: the affected eye is strongly adducted.

The trochlear nerve (Fig. 9b.16) is the only cranial nerve which emerges from the dorsal side of the brain stem. The trochlear nerve originates from the midbrain just caudal to the inferior colliculus of the tectum. It traverses the ambient cistern around the midbrain and enters the dura mater where the tentorial notch attaches to the posterior clinoid process. On most occasions the nerve enters the dura about 1 cm caudal to the posterior clinoid process. The trochlear nerve runs along the roof of the cavernous sinus, passing through the superior orbital fissure into the orbit. It supplies the superior oblique muscle, which rotates the eye downward and laterally. A lesion of the trochlear nerve allows the antagonist muscles to rotate the eye upward and medially.

The oculomotor nerve (Fig. 9b.11) is the largest of the three nerves for the extrinsic ocular muscles. It supplies the remaining four extraocular muscles and the levator palpebrae superioris muscle. In addition, the oculomotor nerve carries parasympathetic fibers for the sphincter pupillae and the ciliary muscles. The oculomotor nerve emerges from the interpeduncular fossa, passes through the similarly named cistern and runs between the superior cerebellar artery and the posterior cerebral artery toward the cavernous sinus. There it runs in the lateral wall of the cavernous sinus and leaves the middle cranial fossa through the superior orbital fissure.

The trigeminal or fifth cranial nerve (Fig. 8b.10) arises from the lateral edge of the pons. It emerges from the posterior cranial fossa and reaches the trigeminal cave in the middle cranial fossa. This flat dural pouch (Meckel's cave) is lined with arachnoid. The trigeminal ganglion (Gasserian or semilunar ganglion) is found here and contains pseudounipolar neurons for the sensory root of the trigeminal nerve. Beyond the ganglion, the trigeminal nerve divides into three large branches: the ophthalmic, maxillary, and mandibular nerves. These branches emerge from the middle cranial fossa through the superior orbital fissure, the foramen rotundum, and foramen ovale, respectively. For the most part, the trigeminal nerve transmits afferent signals from the skin of the face, the conjunctiva and cornea, the mucosa of the nasal and oral cavities, and the teeth. The afferent fibers from the muscle spindles of the muscles of mastication are interconnected in a special way in the trigeminal system (Chap. 4.1.3).

The motor fibers of the trigeminal nerve lie in the medial portion of the nerve and project towards the mandibular nerve. The motor fibers innervate the muscles of mastication, the tensor tympani muscle, and the majority of the muscles of the floor of the mouth.

According to neurosurgical findings, the superior cerebellar artery can compress the trigeminal nerve and may cause trigeminal neuralgia (103, 135, 261).

The optic or second cranial nerve (Figs. 7b.2 and 8b.5) enters the middle cranial fossa through the optic canal. The topography of the optic nerve is described further in Chapter 4.6 (visual system).

The olfactory or first cranial nerve projects through the cribriform plate into the anterior cranial fossa. It is described in detail in Chapter 4.7 (olfactory system).

The topography of the cranial nerves, in relation to each other and to structures at the skull base as well as to blood vessels and to different parts of the human brain, is of considerable clinical relevance. Lesions, that simultaneously affect several cranial nerves, can aid in locating an injury in relation to the course of these nerves. This may be the case with an inflammation or a tumor at the skull base or of the brain itself.

Garcin's syndrome is characterized by a lesion of the caudal cranial nerves, namely the fifth, seventh through twelfth cranial nerves on one side of the skull base.

The jugular foramen syndrome includes disorders of the glossopharyngeal nerve with sensory impairment, frequent pain indicating glossopharyngeal neuralgia and paresis of the soft palate, lesions of the vagus nerve with vocal cord palsy, and unilateral paralysis of the accessory and hypoglossal nerves. Such cases involving concurrent pressure on the medulla oblongata and a resultant contralateral hemiparesis are referred to as Vernet's syndrome.

The cerebellopontine angle syndrome is a disorder of the fifth, seventh, and eighth cranial nerves. Sensory impairment (including loss of the corneal reflex) and/or pain in the facial regions, peripheral facial paresis, and unilateral acoustic and vestibular defects are to be expected. In advanced cases, cerebellar involvement may cause ipsilateral ataxia, nystagmus and occasionally paresis of the abducens nerve may be found.

Gradenigo's syndrome or syndrome of the apex of the petrous bone is marked by unilateral paresis of the abducens nerve and by disorders of the trigeminal nerve with sensory impairment or facial pain, especially in the forehead. Larger lesions may also cause peripheral facial paralysis.

The cavernous sinus syndrome involves a disorder of the three ocular nerves, the third, fourth, and sixth cranial nerves, as well as the trigeminal nerve.

If, in addition to the three ocular cranial nerves, only the first trigeminal branch is affected, a syndrome of the superior orbital fissure is present. Additional presence of unilateral headaches, especially in the temporal region and a non-pulsating exophthalmos, indicate a syndrome of the sphenoid wing. The cause is frequently a meningioma in this region.

A disorder of the third, fourth, sixth, and first branch of the fifth (ophthalmic nerve) cranial nerve with an involvement of the optic nerve is referred to as the orbital apex syndrome. Frequently, the primary symptom is an increasing optic atrophy with corresponding visual impairment.

The olfactory groove syndrome presents first with unilateral and eventually bilateral anosmia. The lesion may also affect the optic nerve, thereby leading to blindness. Large space-occupying lesions, such as meningiomas, are frequently marked by a frontal lobe syndrome with corresponding psychopathological findings.

In the initial stages, lesions responsible for the cranial nerve syndromes located in the region of the skull base are only occasionally seen in CT scans. Supplementary scans made of intermediate sections or additional sectioning planes are often necessary.

3.6 Subdivisions of the Brain

(Figs. 34 and 35)

The brain can be divided into two basic parts:

1. Brain stem together with the cerebellum
2. Forebrain or prosencephalon.

According to international nomenclature the medulla oblongata, pons, and mesencephalon are collectively called the brain stem. The cerebellum is connected to the brain stem by three paired cerebellar peduncles. The forebrain is further divided into the diencephalon and telencephalon. The longitudinal axis of the brain stem (Meynert's axis) and the longitudinal axis of the forebrain (Forel's axis) lie, as mentioned in the introduction (Chap. 1.1), at a 110–120° angle to one another. The axis of the brain stem (Meynert) lies approximately at the floor of the fourth ventricle as a continuation of the caudal portion of the aqueduct. Forel's axis extends from the frontal to the occipital pole of the telencephalon. The angle between the two axes as measured in brains fixed extracranially usually differs from the angle measured in living patients (Chap. 1.2).

3.6.1 Medulla Oblongata and Pons

(Figs. 34 and 35)

The medulla oblongata is a small subdivision of the brain. Its volume is about 7 ml and its basilar surface between the spinal cord and pons is approximately 2 to 2.5 cm long. The area of the cross section through its caudal portion is 1 cm^2 on the average. On the ventral side of the medulla the anterior median fissure continues into the spinal cord. A longitudinal column rises on the medulla oblongata along both sides of the fissure. This paired elevation is called the pyramid. The pyramidal pathway (Chap. 4.8.1) crosses deep within the fissure.

The paired olive-shaped bodies lateral to the pyramids are referred to as olives. The olive contains the inferior olivary nucleus. Nuclear regions of the posterior funiculi form small elevations on the dorsal side of the medulla oblongata. These are called the tubercles of the gracile nucleus (Goll) and cuneate nucleus (Burdach) (52, 190).

Further dorsal portions of the medulla are visible upon removal of the cerebellum along the peduncles (Fig. 36). The fourth ventricle can now be opened. The floor of the rhomboid fossa indicates a continual transition of the medulla oblongata into the pons.

Viewed from a basal direction, the pons is almost twice as wide as the cranial portion of the medulla oblongata. The cranial border of the pons is formed by the cerebral peduncles of the midbrain. Both middle cerebellar peduncles arise from the lateral part of the pons (Fig. 60.14).

The fifth through twelfth cranial nerve nuclei are arranged in a topographical pattern in the medulla and pons (Fig. 36). In the floor of the rhomboid fossa the afferent cranial nerve nuclei lie lateral and the efferent nuclei are located medial. The afferent or sensory nuclei are separated from the efferent nuclei by a weakly developed groove. Two afferent nerves and their sensory nuclei can be seen on the left in Figure 36. On the right the efferent nuclei together with the efferent nerves are illustrated. The sensory nuclei belong to the trigeminal (Chap. 4.1.3), vestibular (Chap. 4.4), auditory (Chap. 4.5), and gustatory (Chap. 4.2) systems. The motor neurons of the fifth, sixth, seventh, ninth, tenth, eleventh, and twelfth cranial nerves lie within the efferent nuclei (Chap. 3.5).

The reticular formation is located as a loose plexus of both large and small nerve cells in the medulla oblongata and pons (122). These nerve cells are polysynaptic, being connected to afferent, efferent, and autonomic systems. The reticular formation is connected as an accessory pathway with afferent systems. Animal experiments have shown that by stimulating the reticular formation the animal may be awakened. Regulatory regions for circulation and respiration are also located in the reticular formation.

Pathways ascending from the anterolateral (Chap. 4.1.1), medial lemniscus (Chap. 4.1.2), trigeminal (Chap. 4.1.3), gustatory (Chap. 4.2), vestibular (Chap. 4.4), and auditory (Chap. 4.5) systems, as well as pathways descending from the motor (Chap. 4.8) and the cerebellar (Chap. 4.9) systems pass through the medulla oblongata and pons.

In canthomeatal parallel planes the medulla oblongata and pons are cut diagonally (at a slight angle to the plane perpendicular to Meynert's axis), so that the resulting sectioning planes lie ventral in a more cranial position and dorsal in a more caudal position than the transverse sections of conventional neuroanatomy books (13, 33, 41, 48, 139, 161, 206,

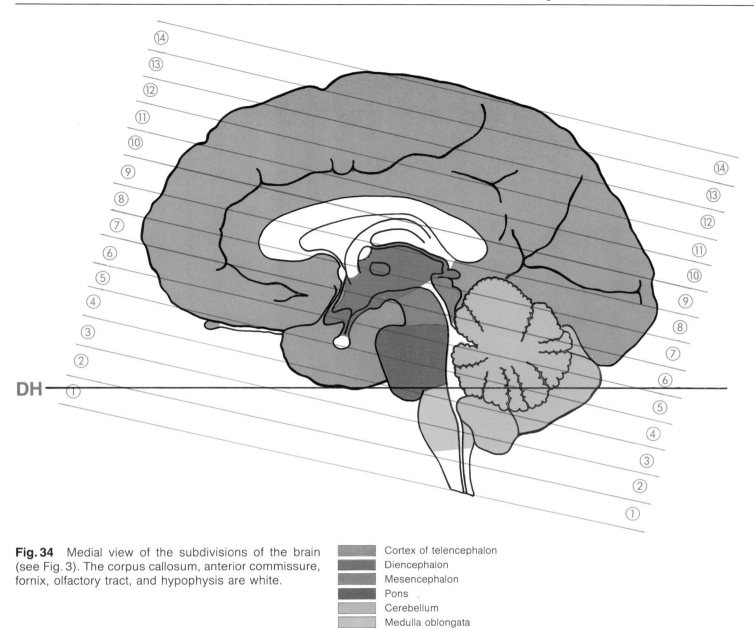

Fig. 34 Medial view of the subdivisions of the brain (see Fig. 3). The corpus callosum, anterior commissure, fornix, olfactory tract, and hypophysis are white.

Cortex of telencephalon
Diencephalon
Mesencephalon
Pons
Cerebellum
Medulla oblongata

245, 269, 283, 318). Typical of this phenomenon is the sectioning plane of the third slice (Fig. 7b), which is located at the border region between the pons and medulla oblongata. In Figure 7 the ventral portion of the pons is cut. The medulla oblongata follows underneath the pons, the dorsal portion being cut almost at the end of the rhomboid fossa. Lying between pons and medulla oblongata, a blind canal (known as foramen cecum) indicates the cranial end of the anterior median fissure of the medulla oblongata. The medulla oblongata can also be seen in Figure 6b and the pons in Figures 8b.13 and 9b.18.

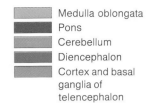

- Medulla oblongata
- Pons
- Cerebellum
- Diencephalon
- Cortex and basal ganglia of telencephalon

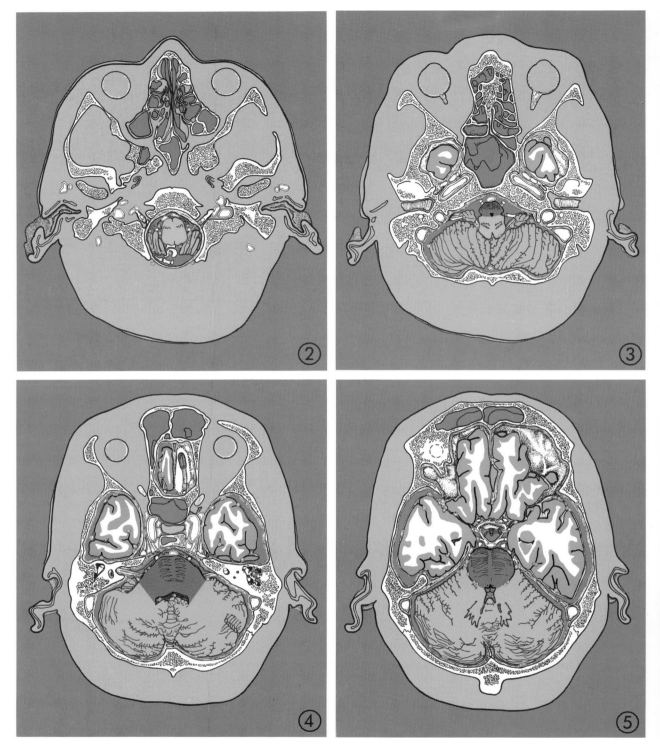

Fig. 35 Serial illustrations of the subdivisions of the brain. The encircled number indicates the number of the slice (see Figs. 1a, 2, 3, 4).

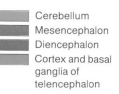

Cerebellum
Mesencephalon
Diencephalon
Cortex and basal ganglia of telencephalon

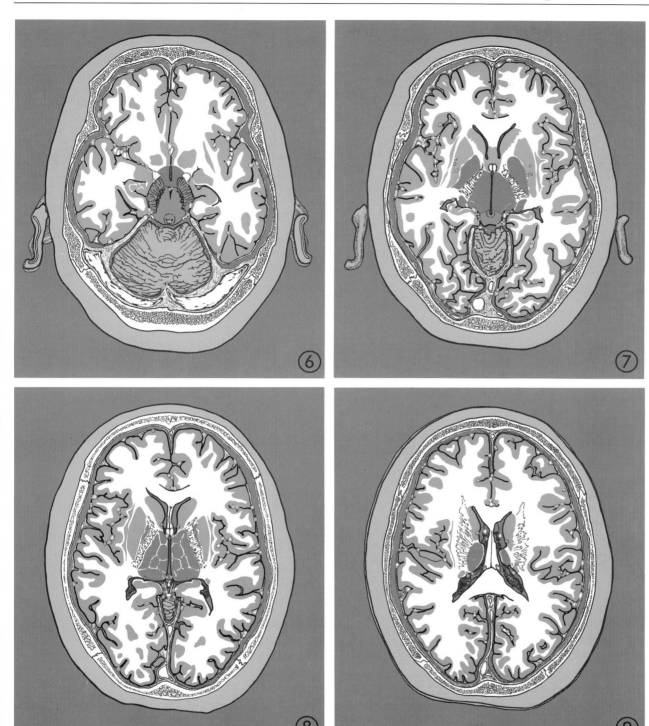

Cortex of
telencephalon

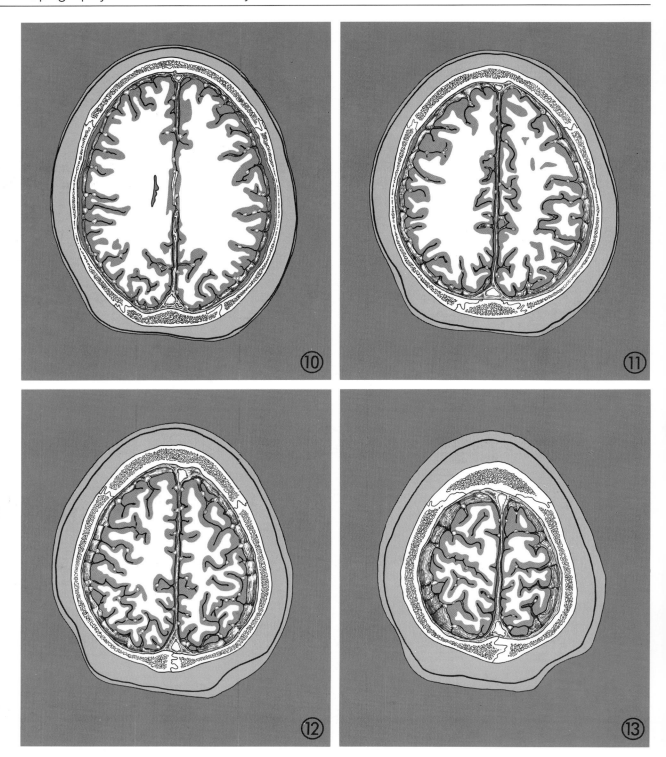

Fig. 35 Serial illustrations of the subdivisions of the
brain. The encircled number indicates the number of
the slice (see Figs. 1a, 2, 3, 4).

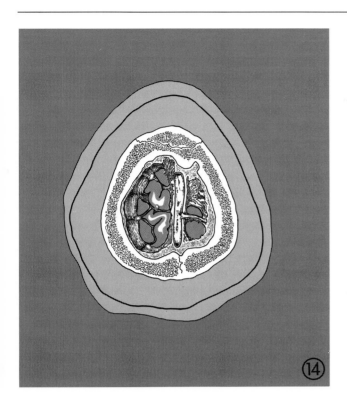

Lesions of the medulla oblongata and pons frequently affect the cranial nerve nuclei and their connections with one another as well as their connections with the spinal cord, cerebellum, and cerebrum. The efferent and afferent pathways between the cerebrum or more specifically, between the basal efferent ganglia and spinal cord, are affected simultaneously. Small foci lead to ipsilateral disorders of the caudal cranial nerves and to contralateral paresis of the extremities and/or sensory impairment. Clinically recognizable symptoms usually suffice in localizing the damage and identifying the type of brain stem syndrome. The different syndromes are seldom described with any consistency and clinically rarely present in their pure form. One of the most common syndromes is the Wallenberg's syndrome showing acute symptoms like rotatory vertigo, nausea and vomiting, and hoarseness. Examination reveals nystagmus, ipsilateral Horner's syndrome, trigeminal disorder, palate and rear pharyngeal wall paresis, and hemiataxia of the extremities. A dissociated sensory loss of the extremities and the trunk exists contralaterally.

Extensive lesions cause a bulbar paralysis with tetraplegia. Smaller lesions are seldom evident in CT scans. The main causes of Wallenberg's syndrome are ischemia, especially in the medulla oblongata, and bleeding and/or the presence of tumors in the pons. Foci in cases of multiple sclerosis should also be considered.

1 Mesencephalic tract of trigeminal nerve
2 Mesencephalic nucleus of trigeminal nerve
3 Main sensory (pontine) nucleus of trigeminal nerve
4 Spinal tract of trigeminal nerve
5 Spinal nucleus of trigeminal nerve
6 Vestibular nuclei
7 Cochlear nuclei
8 Solitary nucleus
9 Accessory oculomotor nucleus (Edinger-Westphal)
10 Oculomotor nucleus
11 Trochlear nucleus
12 Motor nucleus of trigeminal nerve
13 Genu of facial nerve
14 Abducens nucleus
15 Facial nucleus
16 Salivatory nuclei
17 Nucleus ambiguus
18 Dorsal nucleus of vagus nerve
19 Hypoglossal nucleus
20 Spinal nucleus of accessory nerve

Vm Motor root of trigeminal nerve

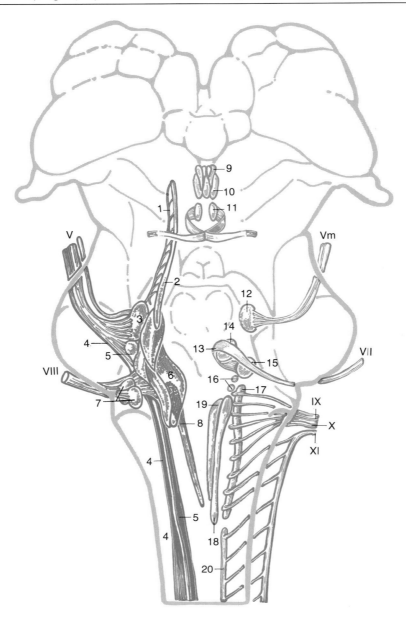

Fig. 36 Cranial nerve nuclei III-XII in the spinal cord, medulla oblongata, pons, and mesencephalon. The left side illustrates the sensory nuclei with two afferent nerves and fiber bundles. On the right there are the motor and parasympathetic nuclei with efferent nerves. Roman numerals indicate the cranial nerves. According to (206).

3.6.2 Cerebellum (Figs. 34, 35, 59)

The cerebellum is divided into a narrow median zone, the vermis, and two hemispheres. The primary fissure (Fig. 10b.41) separates the anterior lobe of the cerebellum from the posterior lobe. The anterior lobe (Figs. 10b.38, 10b.39, 11b.41) is part of the paleocerebellum; the posterior lobe, excluding the pyramis of vermis and the uvula of vermis, is part of the neocerebellum. The flocculus (Fig. 7b.12) and nodule of vermis belong to the archeocerebellum. The cerebellar peduncles reflect the paleoneo-cerebellar arrangements (Fig. 60). Afferent systems project via the inferior and superior cerebellar peduncles to the paleocerebellum (Figs. 60.6 and 60.13). The middle cerebellar peduncle connects the neocortex with the neocerebellum via the pontine nuclei (Fig. 60.14).

The cerebellum has a thin cortex of gray matter (approximately 1 mm thick). In the white matter from lateral to medial, lie the following paired cerebellar nuclei: dentate, emboliform, globose, and fastigial nuclei. The afferent and efferent cerebellar pathways are described in Chapter 4.9 (cerebellar systems).

The cerebellum fills most of the infratentorial space. On the average the cerebellum has a volume of 150 ml in males and 135 ml in females (249, 316). The relatively large portion of the infratentorial space occupied by the cerebellum compared to that occupied by the medulla oblongata and pons is clearly evident in Figure 35.

The tonsils of cerebellum reach furthest into the posterior cranial fossa and are thereby the most caudal portion of the cerebellum (Fig. 6b.9). The posterior lobe is located cranial to the tonsils. The flocculus (Fig. 7b.12) lies in the cerebellopontine (angle) cistern (Fig. 27.6). As seen in canthomeatal serial illustrations, the anterior lobe is the part located most cranial (Figs. 10b.38, 10b.39, 11b.41, 12b.41).

Cerebellar lesions are characterized by dyssynergias (disturbances of muscular coordination with ataxia, postural anomalies, and speech impairment), by hypotonia (decreased muscle tone), and by a disturbance of equilibrium. Archeocerebellar lesions resulting in an impairment of the transmission of vestibular signals cause equilibrium disorders as well as trunk and gait ataxia. Lesions of the neocerebellum cause an ipsilateral impairment of movement in the extremities with ataxia, intention tremor, and dysdiadochokinesia. A frequent additional cerebellar symptom is nystagmus.

3.6.3 Mesencephalon (Figs. 34 and 35)

The mesencephalon or midbrain is a small division of the brain with a volume of about 10 ml. The base of the mesencephalon is approximately 1.5 cm long. At the tectum it has a length of 2 cm. The midbrain can be divided into three levels, which are oriented in the transverse plane around the aqueduct. The roof of the midbrain is called the tectum (tectal lamina, quadrigeminal plate). The tegmentum of the cerebral peduncle lies in the middle of the midbrain. The basal portion of the midbrain is formed by the base of the cerebral peduncle (crura cerebri). The aqueduct ascends in a concave curve between the fourth and third ventricles. Transverse sections through the midbrain, which are cut perpendicular to the aqueduct, cannot, therefore, be parallel to each other. Histological serial sections through a block of midbrain tissue can be made against either the cranial or caudal transverse plane of the aqueduct. For this reason, transverse serial sections through the midbrain vary greatly (13, 33, 41, 48, 139, 161, 206, 269, 283, 318). Furthermore, these transverse midbrain sections differ from those made parallel to the canthomeatal plane (Fig. 3). In the brain illustrated, the sectioning plane runs through the midbrain at an obtuse angle; the ventral part of the cerebral peduncle is cut more cranially, the dorsal part (tectum) more caudally. In Figure 12a the superior colliculi are concealed beneath the internal cerebral vein (Fig. 12a.12) and the great cerebral vein (Galen) (Fig. 12a.19). In Figure 11b the inferior colliculi are visible (Fig. 11b.39). The cerebral peduncle lies inside the seventh slice and, therefore, cannot be seen. The base of the cerebral peduncle is depicted in Figure 10b.28. Midbrains taken from those brains used for comparison were not cut as flat as the one illustrated in this book. After CT and anatomic studies it was recommended to examine the midbrain in an approximately infraorbitomeatal parallel plane (17). CT images obtained in this plane resemble more closely those of known transverse sections of the midbrain. Furthermore, CT examination of the interpeduncular cistern, ambient cistern, and cistern of the tectal lamina, along with their contents, is better done in the infraorbitomeatal plane than in the canthomeatal plane.

The tectum of the midbrain is a thin plate marked by four roundish elevations. The two caudal elevations, the inferior colliculi, are lower and narrower than the superior colliculi. The inferior colliculi are relay stations for the auditory system. The superior colliculi, on the other hand, serve as a visual reflex center. From here, the short tectobulbar tract and long tectospinal tract descend to motor neurons in the brain stem and spinal cord.

The tegmentum of the midbrain contains the motor nuclei of the third and fourth cranial nerves

(Figs. 36.9, 36.10, 36.11). The medial and most cranial located parasympathetic accessory oculomotor nucleus (Edinger-Westphal) innervates the sphincter pupillae muscle (miosis) and the ciliary muscle (accommodation). The root fibers of the third cranial nerve project basally through the red nucleus and emerge at the interpeduncular fossa. The motor nucleus of the fourth cranial nerve lies caudal to the nucleus of the oculomotor nerve. The root fibers of the trochlear nerve extend dorsally, cross over, and leave the tectum caudal to the inferior colliculi (Fig. 36). Dorsolateral to these motor nuclei lies the mesencephalic nucleus of the trigeminal nerve (Chap. 4.1.3).

The reticular formation constitutes the framework of the tegmentum. Structure and function of the reticular formation have been described in connection with the medulla oblongata and pons on page 80. The red nucleus and the substantia nigra, which are considered as parts of the basal ganglia (Chap. 4.8.2), are located in the tegmentum of the midbrain. The red nucleus, a short cigar-shaped structure, extends from the tegmentum to the diencephalon. The characteristic black color of the substantia nigra, a plate of nerve cells located in the basal portion of the midbrain (Fig. 10b.29), is due to the high concentration of melanin found in its nerve cells. The axons of these dopaminergic neurons (A 9) project into the striatum. This nigrostriate system is described in Chapter 4.12.1 (dopaminergic systems).

The paired base of the cerebral peduncles contains only descending pathways from the neocortex. These pathways as seen in medial to lateral direction are:

- Frontopontine tract
- Motor cranial nerve pathway or corticonuclear tract
- Pyramidal pathway or corticospinal tract
- Occipitotemporopontine tract.

The frontopontine and occipitotemporopontine tracts are part of the cerebellar system (Chap. 4.9). The corticonuclear and corticospinal tracts are part of the pyramidal system (Chap. 4.8.1).

The ascending pathways run through the tegmentum. The medial lemniscus system (Chap. 4.1.2) lies dorsolateral to the red nucleus. The fibers of the anterolateral and trigeminal systems lie close to the medial lemniscus. Located further lateral is the lateral lemniscus, a part of the auditory system (Chap. 4.5).

Mesencephalic dysfunctions are characterized by paralysis of vertical gaze, paresis of the eye muscles controlled by the third and fourth cranial nerves, and by ataxia and, occasionally, tremor. Injuries to the reticular formation and oral mesencephalic structures, as well as to those structures localized in the border region between the midbrain and diencephalon can cause akinetic mutism. Such dysfunctions often develop posttraumatically.

3.6.4 Diencephalon (Figs. 34 and 35)

The diencephalon encircles the third ventricle and is bordered by the mesencephalon and telencephalon. It consists of nuclear regions traversed by fiber bundles.

As mentioned earlier, the shift of the longitudinal axis of the forebrain (Forel's axis) during evolution of the neuronal systems of the neocortex forced the nuclear regions of the human diencephalon into new topographical positions. Many of these diencephalic nuclear regions were first described in mammals, in which the neocortex is not as highly developed. The names given in comparative anatomy to the nuclear diencephalic regions did not change in human neuroanatomy. Thus, when referring to the positions of the subnuclei of the human diencephalon, directional descriptions like "ventral" and "dorsal" are only correct relative to Forel's axis and do not correspond to the long axis of the human body. This inconsistency in nomenclature is especially obvious in the illustrations of the forebrain made in the canthomeatal parallel planes, as in serial sections of the whole head the anatomical position can be easily identified by the frontal (ventral) and occipital (dorsal) part of the skull.

Arranged in a caudal to cranial sequence, the illustrations of the diencephalon first show only the hypothalamus and its infundibulum (Fig. 9b.9). In the next illustration, the hypothalamus (Fig. 10b.17) and telencephalic lamina terminalis are visible (Fig. 10b.16). The subsequent illustrations depict the hypothalamus (Fig. 11b.22), thalamic parts (Fig. 11b.30), metathalamus (Figs. 11b.31 and 11b.32), and globus pallidus (Figs. 11b.14 and 11b.15). In Figure 12, the next parallel plane, the subnuclei of the thalamus with the habenular nuclei (Figs. 12b.23-28), and the globus pallidus (Fig. 12b.18) are seen. The last and most cranial section of the series shows only the thalamus (Fig. 13b.18). With occasional exceptions, the diencephalon is divided in a caudal to cranial direction into the following parts:

- Hypothalamus
- Subthalamus and globus pallidus
- Metathalamus
- Thalamus
- Epithalamus.

The hypothalamus forms the base of the diencephalon. It surrounds the funnel-shaped caudal portion of the third ventricle that extends caudally into the infundibular recess. The infundibulum connects the hypothalamus with the pituitary gland. The hypothalamus borders rostrally on the lamina terminalis (Fig. 10b.16) and the anterior commissure. The optic chiasm is located basal to the hypothalamus (Fig. 9b.8). Dorsal to the infundibulum lie the tuber cinereum and mamillary bodies. The hypothalamic sulcus forms the border on the wall of the third ventricle between the hypothalamus and thalamus. The hypothalamus laterally reaches the subthalamic nucleus.

Morphologically and functionally, the hypothalamus is closely connected with the hypophysis or pituitary gland. The axonal fibers of the neurosecretory cells in the hypothalamus project through the infundibulum into the neurohypophysis or posterior lobe of the hypophysis. These neurosecretory cells produce the neurohypophyseal hormones oxytocin and vasopressin (ADH, antidiuretic hormone). Damage to this hypothalamic-neurohypophyseal system results in diabetes insipidus. The adenohypophysis or anterior lobe of the pituitary gland is connected to the hypothalamus through the hypophyseal portal system. The hypothalamic-infundibular system produces substances that either trigger the release of hormones in the anterior lobe of the pituitary gland (releasing factors, RF) or inhibit the secretion of hypophyseal hormones (inhibiting factors, IF). It is presumed that this system is controlled by the tuberoinfundibular dopaminergic system (Chap. 4.12.1).

The hypothalamus can be divided according to its content of myelinated nerve fibers into a strongly myelinated hypothalamus and a weakly myelinated hypothalamus. The nerve cells of the hypothalamic-neurohypophyseal system, the hypothalamic-infundibular system and non-hypophyseal nerve cells are part of the weakly myelinated hypothalamus. The non-hypophyseal nerve cells are located, for the most part, in the lateral regions of the hypothalamus and control autonomic activities such as regulation of body temperature, food and water intake, sleep, and emotional behavior. The nuclear groups in the mamillary body are part of the strongly myelinated hypothalamus. Morphologically and functionally, these groups are closely related to the limbic system (Chap. 4.11).

The subthalamus and metathalamus are located in the lateral portion of the diencephalon but do not come into contact with the wall of the third ventricle. The subthalamic nucleus represents the major portion of the subthalamus. This nucleus lies dorsal to the mamillary body and medial to the internal capsule and is located deep in the seventh slice (Fig. 58.7). Located in the vicinity of the subthalamic nucleus but lateral to the internal capsule is the globus pallidus (Fig. 11b.14, 11b.15, 12b.18). It is considered part of the basal ganglia and is involved in motor activities (Chap. 4.8.2).

The metathalamus consists of the medial and lateral geniculate bodies (Figs. 11b.31 and 11b.32) which are located dorsal to the thalamus. The medial geniculate body is a relay nucleus for the auditory system (Chap. 4.5), while the lateral geniculate body is a relay center for the visual system (Chap. 4.6).

The thalamus is a somewhat egg-shaped aggregate of numerous nuclear regions. The tip of this "egg" is directed toward the interventricular foramen (Monro) (Fig. 12b.22). The medial surface of the thalamus borders on the third ventricle. Its lateral surface contacts the posterior limb of the internal capsule (Fig. 12b.20). The dorsal portion of the thalamus (Fig. 12b.28) is the pulvinar. The interthalamic adhesion (intermediate mass) (Fig. 3.15), a narrow bridge of glia cells, usually connects the thalami of both sides. A narrow portion of the superior side of the thalamus develops embryonally into the floor of the central part of the lateral ventricle. This area is called the lamina affixa and would appear in Figure 13b.18 just above the visible portion of the thalamus. Lateral to the thalamus lies the caudate nucleus (Figs. 13b.12 and 13b.22). The thalamostriate vein (Fig. 13a.11) and the stria terminalis run in the groove between these two nuclear regions.

Medullary laminae divide the nuclear complexes of the thalamus into several groups. In the rostral portion of the thalamus two laminae separate the anterior thalamic nuclei (Fig. 12b.23). These nuclei are, for the most part, relay stations of the limbic system (Chap. 4.11). Medially, an internal lamina forms the border of a medial nuclear group, one nucleus being the medial thalamic nucleus (Fig. 12b.24). The medial nucleus has corticopedal and corticofugal connections with the frontal lobe of the telencephalon.

Of the many lateral nuclei of the thalamus, only those which are of special importance to the neurofunctional systems will be described. In general, the thalamic nuclei have both thalamocortical and corticothalamic fibers, although often only one projectional system may be mentioned.

Stereotactic surgery can be performed on several of the relay nuclei. The common clinical synonyms for such nuclei are given in parentheses along with the international name (105, 107, 264, 265, 266). The ventral lateral nucleus (nucleus ventrooralis (107)) (Fig. 12b.25) is connected with area 4 (located rostral to the central sulcus in the frontal lobe). The frontal portion of the ventral lateral nucleus contains afferent fibers from the internal pallidum, while the occipital portion contains afferent fibers from the cerebellum. The ventral posterolateral nucleus (nucleus ventrocaudalis externus (107)) (Fig. 11b.30) is a relay nucleus for the anterolateral and the medial lemniscus systems. In its immediate vicinity lies the ventral posteromedial nucleus (nucleus ventrocaudalis internus (107)) (Fig. 45.3). This nucleus provides a similar relay center for the trigeminal system with a somatotopic projection into the postcentral gyrus as does its neighboring nucleus (Chap. 4.1.3). The ventral posterolateral and posteromedial nuclei belong to the specific nuclei of the thalamus. They have point-to-point connections with the body periphery and specific areas of the cerebral cortex.

The mode of connection of these specific nuclei is different from that of the nonspecific nuclei that project diffusely into large areas of the telencephalon. The intralaminar nuclei, as described in Chapter 4.3 (ascending reticular system), belong to these nonspecific nuclei. The pulvinar transmits both auditory and optic signals and projects into secondary cortical areas of the telencephalon.

The epithalamus is composed of structures located on and around the roof of the third ventricle. These structures include the choroid plexus of the third ventricle, the stria medullaris thalami, the habenular nuclei (Fig. 12b.27), and the pineal gland (pineal body, epiphysis) (Fig. 12a.18). Just ventral to the superior colliculi lies the posterior commissure (Fig. 3.18), which joins nuclear groups of the midbrain. The pineal gland, which has an average length of slightly less than 1 cm, lies on the tectum and is attached to the roof of the diencephalon. In about 10% of school children examined, acervulus is found in the pineal gland. After the age of twenty-five, CT scans reveal that pineal gland calcifications increase to more than 50% (320). These calcifications are a CT guideline structure indicating the position of the pineal gland.

Diencephalic lesions result in characteristic dysfunctions which, in certain cases, enable a topical assessment after clinical examination. A "central" dysregulation of body temperature or disorders of fluid balance, for instance, indicate hypothalamic or, more specifically, hypothalamic-neurohypophyseal dysfunction. Other symptoms indicating hypothalamic dysfunction are severe impairments of sympathetic/parasympathetic regulatory functions.

The subthalamus is in close contact with the basal ganglia via the globus pallidus. A lesion in this region results in contralateral hemiballism. A vascular disorder is the most frequent cause.

Depending on the anatomical location, thalamic dysfunctions may take on many forms. The thalamus is not only a subcortical collection point for exteroceptive and proprioceptive impulses (62), but also a relay station for optic and auditory pathways, as well as an important integration and coordination center for afferent impulses and their affective influences. Lesions cause contralateral disorders of both exteroceptive sensitivity, especially thermal sense and proprioceptive sensitivity. Patients develop hemiataxia and involuntary movements as well as choreoathetoid movements. Contralateral spontaneous pain and hyperpathia may arise. Thalamic disorders can often be traced to vascular causes. Tumors seldom cause a complete thalamic syndrome.

A unilateral lesion of the medial geniculate body usually remains undetected because of the bilateral nature of the auditory pathway. A unilateral injury of the lateral geniculate body, on the other hand, leads to a contralateral visual field defect up to a homonymous contralateral hemianopsia.

3.6.5 Telencephalon
(Figs. 34, 35, 37, 38, 39)

The telencephalon or endbrain consists of telencephalic nuclei, the olfactory bulb and tract, and the brain mantle or pallium. Averaging more than 1000 ml, the telencephalon is the largest subdivision of the brain. As it makes up more than 80% of the total volume of the brain, the supratentorial space is predominantly filled with telencephalic structures. As seen in the illustrations, the upper canthomeatal parallel planes depict nothing but portions of the telencephalon (Fig. 35). In the lower parallel canthomeatal planes, the telencephalon reaches as far as the fourth slice, extending into the anterior cranial fossa as the olfactory bulb and tract (Figs. 8b.3 and 8b.4). The base of the temporal lobe (Fig. 7b.3), the most basal portion of the telencephalon, reaches into the middle cranial fossa and lies almost directly above the canthomeatal plane in the third slice.

The external form of the telencephalon is marked by the two hemispheres. The interhemispheric fissure separates the two hemispheres in the median plane down to the corpus callosum. Stretching between the hemispheres is a dural septum, the cerebral falx (Figs. 10b.3, 11b.3, 12b.3, 13b.3, 14b.3, 15b.14, 16b.10, 17b.7). The medial surface of each hemisphere lies parallel to the median plane. The superior margin marks the area of each hemisphere, where the medial surface meets the lateral surface. The lateral surface of the human telencephalon is formed entirely by the neocortex. During evolution, its surface area increased through the development of convolutions or gyri and furrows or sulci. Located beneath the cortex are corticopetal, corticofugal, and intercortical pathways. They form the white matter of the telencephalon. The nuclei of the telencephalon border on the lateral ventricles. These nuclei have been divided by the ascending and descending neencephalic pathways into the following formations:

- Caudate nucleus (Figs. 11b.16, 11b.33, 12b.10, 12b.34, 13b.12, 13b.22)
- Putamen (Figs. 11b.13 and 12b.17)
- Claustrum (Figs. 10b.13, 11b.11, 12b.15, 13b.13)
- Amygdaloid body (nucleus) (Figs. 9b.12 and 10b.21)
- Septum verum (Fig. 11b.20).

During evolution of the neocortex, the caudate nucleus assumed the shape of an arched tail contoured along the wall of the lateral ventricle. The head of the caudate nucleus is a relatively large bulging protuberance on the lateral wall of the anterior horn of the lateral ventricle. It continues occipitally along this wall as the body of the caudate nucleus, then turning rostrally in the roof of the lateral ventricle, where it forms the tail of the caudate nucleus. This tail tapers to a point in the roof of the temporal horn. Neencephalic pathways separate the caudate nucleus from the putamen with the exception of those parts located in the rostrobasal region (floor of the striatum, Fig. 10b.12). As the nerve cells of both nuclear regions are similar in form and function, the caudate nucleus and putamen are referred to as striatum. The striatum has an important motor function (Chap. 4.8.2).

The putamen is a shell-shaped structure located medial to the external capsule. The globus pallidus of the diencephalon lies inside the concave portion of the putamen. Topographically, the putamen and globus pallidus form the lentiform nucleus. The nerve cells of these two nuclear regions, however, differ substantially.

The claustrum lies as a small plate-like structure lateral to the putamen and is bordered on opposite sides by the external and extreme capsules.

The amygdaloid body (amygdala or amygdaloid nucleus) is located in a medial position at the tip of the temporal horn of the lateral ventricle. One part of the amygdaloid body belongs to the olfactory system (Chap. 4.7), the other part to the limbic system (Chap. 4.11).

The septum verum (precommissural septum) is a nuclear region located cranial to the anterior commissure and frontal to the column of the fornix. It is described further in Chapter 4.11 as part of the limbic system.

The olfactory bulb lies on the cribriform plate in the anterior cranial fossa (Fig. 8b.3). It receives the olfactory nerves from the olfactory epithelium in the upper posterior part of the nasal cavity. The fibers of the olfactory tract (Fig. 8b.4) project via the medial and lateral olfactory striae to the olfactory cortex, which is located in the gyrus semilunaris and in the cortical regions of the amygdaloid body (Chap. 4.7).

The brain mantle or pallium, which consists of the cerebral cortex and the white matter beneath it, encloses the lateral ventricles. The pallium is divided into four lobes and the insula which has been covered by the opercula during evolution of the neocortex (Figs. 37–39):

● Frontal lobe
● Parietal lobe
● Occipital lobe
● Temporal lobe
● Insula or island of Reil.

The individual lobes are only partially separated by sulci. Located on the lateral surface of each hemisphere, the central sulcus (Figs. 12b.29, 13b.11, 14b.7, 15b.4, 16b.5, 17b.4, 18b.2) separates the frontal lobe from the parietal lobe. The lateral sulcus (Sylvian fissure) (Figs. 10b.7, 11b.25, 12b.12) forms the boundary of the temporal lobe against the frontal lobe and reaches deep into the brain toward the insula. For a short distance it also separates the temporal and parietal lobes. On the medial surface of each hemisphere, the parieto-occipital sulcus (Figs. 12b.39, 13b.25, 14b.17, 15b.12, 16b.12) divides the parietal and occipital lobes. In the dorsolateral region of the lateral surface of each hemisphere, there are no clear boundaries between the parietal, occipital, and temporal lobes.

The lateral surface of the frontal lobe shows three arched gyri only partially separated by sulci. These are:

● Superior frontal gyrus (Figs. 10b.1, 11b.1, 12b.1, 13b.1, 14b.1, 15b.1, 16b.1, 17b.1)
● Middle frontal gyrus (Figs. 10b.4, 11b.2, 12b.2, 13b.2, 14b.2, 15b.2, 16b.2)
● Inferior frontal gyrus (Figs. 10b.5, 11b.5, 12b.4, 13b.7).

The inferior frontal gyrus is further divided by two ascending branches of the lateral (Sylvian) sulcus. The portion of the frontal gyrus located dorsal to the ascending branch is called frontal operculum. In more than 95% of all individuals, Broca's area (motor language area) is located in this region of the left hemisphere (Chap. 4.10). All three frontal gyri terminate at the precentral sulcus (Figs. 14b.5, 16b.3, 17b.2). Located between the precentral and central sulci is a motor region, the precentral gyrus (Figs. 12b.11, 13b.9, 14b.6, 15b.3, 16b.4, 17b.3, 18b.1). Situated on the medial surface of each hemisphere, the paracentral lobule is a portion of this motor region. Above the roof of the orbit in the anterior cranial fossa lie variable convolutions of the frontal lobe, known as the orbital gyri (Fig. 9b.2). The gyrus rectus (Figs. 8b.2 and 9b.3) is bordered laterally by the olfactory sulcus.

The postcentral gyrus (Figs. 12b.30, 13b.15, 14b.10, 15b.7, 16b.6, 17b.5, 18b.3) of the parietal lobe borders on the central sulcus. The normally fragmentary postcentral sulcus runs dorsally along the postcentral gyrus partitioning off the superior parietal lobule (Figs. 16b.9 and 17b.9). The supramarginal gyrus (Figs. 14b.13 and 15b.9) and the angular gyrus (Figs. 14b.15 and 15b.10) are considered as portions of the parietal lobe. The supramarginal gyrus forms a concave convolution around the posterior end of the lateral sulcus (Sylvian fissure). The angular gyrus curves around the occipital end of the superior temporal sulcus. The precuneus (Figs. 14b.16, 15b.11,

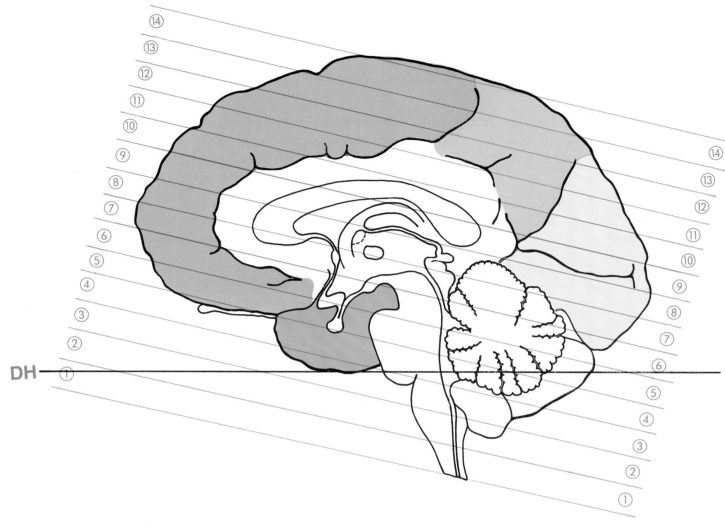

Fig. 37 Medial view of the brain indicating the boundaries of the frontal, parietal, occipital and temporal lobes. The cingulate gyrus with the paraterminal gyrus and the subcallosal area are not considered part of any lobe.

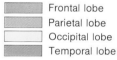
Frontal lobe
Parietal lobe
Occipital lobe
Temporal lobe

16b.11, 17b.10), located on the medial surface of each hemisphere, is considered part of the parietal lobe.

The occipital gyri (Figs. 11b.45, 12b.42, 13b.27, 14b.19) are somewhat irregular-shaped convolutions located on the lateral surface of the occipital lobe. Lying on the caudal surface of the occipital lobe and facing the tentorium of cerebellum are the lateral and medial occipitotemporal gyri (Figs. 11b.42 and 11b.44). Half of these gyri belong to the occipital lobe, half to the temporal lobe. The cuneus (Figs. 13b.26, 14b.20, 15b.15) lies on the medial side of the occipital lobe between the parieto-occipital and calcarine sulci. The crnea on both sides of the calcarine sulcus (Figs. 12b.44 and 53.17) belongs to the primary visual cortex.

The temporal lobe has three temporal gyri:
● Superior temporal gyrus (Figs. 9b.4, 10b.10, 11b.27, 12b.31, 13b.20)
● Middle temporal gyrus (Figs. 9b.6, 10b.22, 11b.38, 12b.38)
● Inferior temporal gyrus (Figs. 8b.8, 9b.17, 10b.32).

These temporal gyri cross Reid's base line at an acute angle (Fig. 38). They are separated by the superior and inferior temporal sulci. Lying in the lateral sulcus between the superior temporal gyrus and the dorsal edge of the insula are the transverse temporal gyri (Heschl) (Figs. 12b.32 and 13b.21). The primary auditory cortex is located here. On the caudal side of the temporal lobe, the lateral and medial occipitotemporal gyri (mentioned above) border on

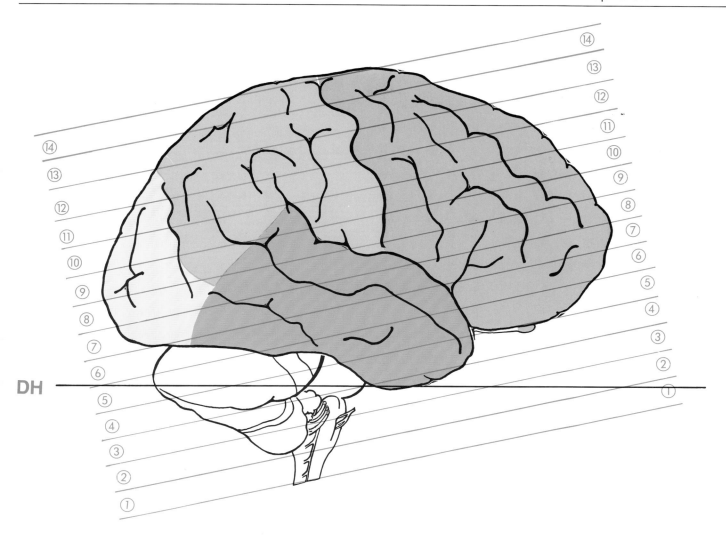

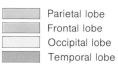

Fig. 38 Lateral view of the brain indicating the boundaries of the frontal, parietal, occipital, and temporal lobes.

- Parietal lobe
- Frontal lobe
- Occipital lobe
- Temporal lobe

the inferior temporal gyrus. Further medial lies the parahippocampal gyrus (Figs. 9b.15, 10b.27, 11b.37) with the hippocampal uncus (Fig. 10b.25). These portions of the temporal lobe belong to the phylogenetically older divisions of the brain. Buried deep in the temporal lobe, the hippocampus borders on the temporal horn of the lateral ventricle (Figs. 10b.24, 11b.36, 12b.37). Together with rudimentary cortical structures on the corpus callosum and a small convolution frontal to the corpus callosum, the hippocampus serves as the internal boundary of the limbic system (Chap. 4.11). The parahippocampal gyrus, the segment of the cingulate gyrus near the corpus callosum (Figs. 10b.6, 11b.4, 12b.5, 13b.5, 14b.8, 15b.6, 63.1), and the subcallosal area surround the corpus callosum and form the external boundary of the limbic system.

The insula lies deep in the lateral sulcus (Figs. 10b.14, 11b.9, 12b.13, 13b.14). It is covered by the frontal, parietal, and temporal portions of the neencephalon. The corresponding gyri are referred to as the frontal, parietal, and temporal opercula. The insula contains the visceral areas.

Located on the medial surface of the brain is a group of gyri that form a boundary along the corpus callosum. This boundary extends without interruption throughout the separate cerebral lobes (Fig. 37), and, for this reason, the subcallosal area and the cingulate gyrus are not considered part of any cerebral lobe.

When observed from a caudal to cranial direction, the parallel canthomeatal planes initially show the basal surface of the temporal lobe lying in the middle cranial fossa (Fig. 39, third slice). In the fourth slice,

Cortex of
temporal lobe

Cortex of
frontal lobe

Cortex of
occipital lobe

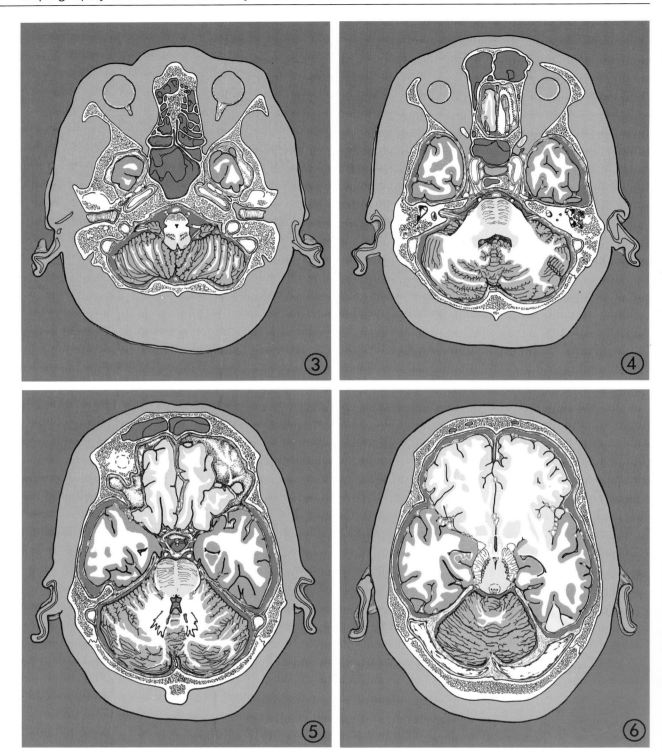

Fig. 39 Serial illustrations of the cortices of the frontal, parietal, occipital, and temporal lobes. The cortices of the insula, cingulate gyrus, subcallosal area, and paraterminal gyrus are not considered part of any lobe. The encircled number indicates the number of the respective slice (see Figs. 1a, 2, 3, 4).

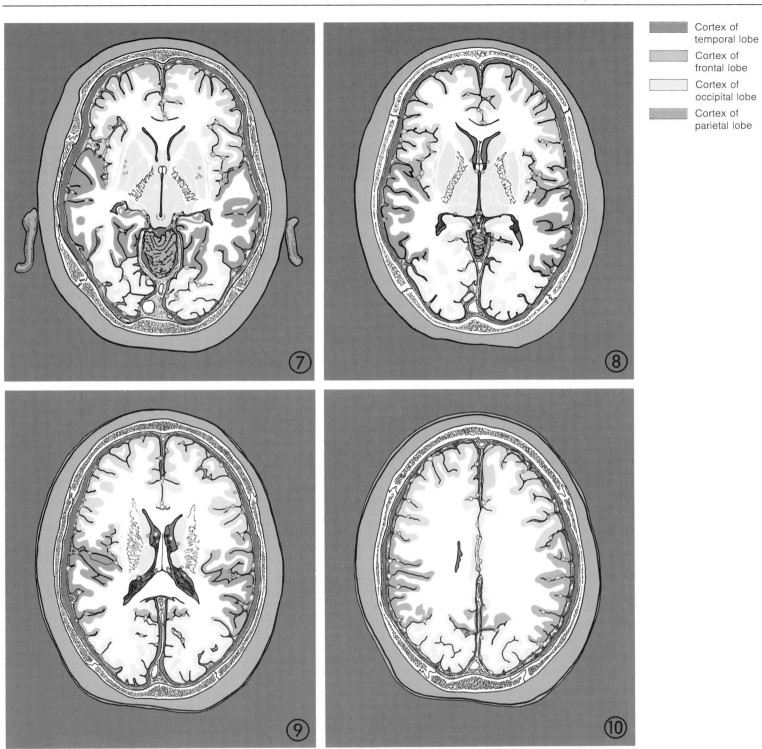

Cortex of
temporal lobe

Cortex of
frontal lobe

Cortex of
occipital lobe

Cortex of
parietal lobe

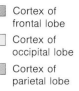

Cortex of
frontal lobe

Cortex of
occipital lobe

Cortex of
parietal lobe

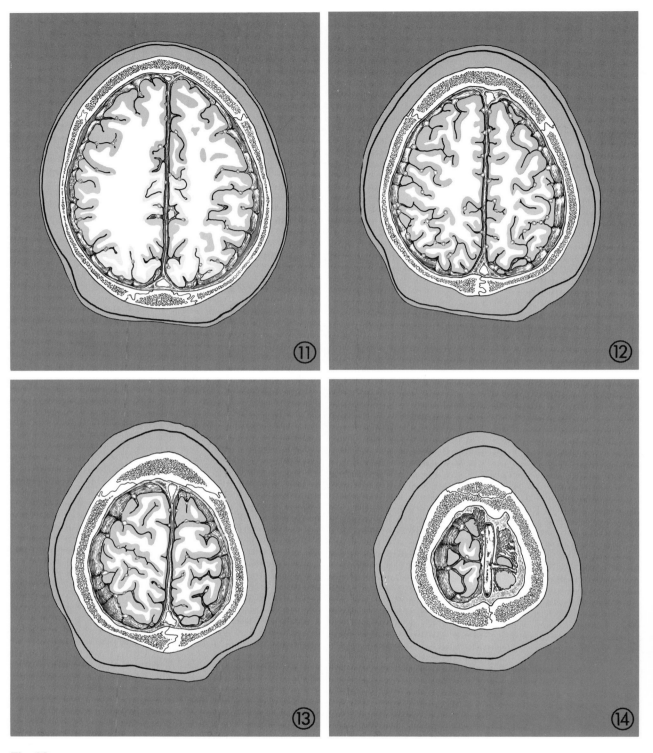

Fig. 39

one centimeter higher, the sectioning plane cuts through the recess in the anterior cranial fossa, the cribriform plate. The olfactory bulb and tract, as well as basal portions of the frontal lobe, are located in this recess. The cross-sectional areas of the frontal and temporal lobes increase in the fifth and sixth slices. At the level of the lateral ventricle, the occipital and parietal lobes do appear. In the ninth slice, the frontal, parietal, temporal, and occipital lobes interdigitate. The temporal lobe does not extend into the supraventricular area. The two most superior slices contain parts of the frontal and parietal lobes only.

Four exemplary CT images of the head are provided in Figures 40a–d. The anatomical sections depicted in Figures 5 to 18 are taken from the same head. The CT scans were made post mortem after formalin-alcohol fixation of the brain (Chap. 1.3). The scans were taken at the levels of the eighth, ninth, tenth, and twelfth slices. They illustrate the diencephalic-telencephalic region of the brain. Intracranially trapped air, which produces a spotty accentuation of the external CSF spaces, greatly impairs the quality of these CT images.

It should be noted that the subarachnoid space appears disproportionately large as a result of the shrinkage of the brain tissue. The relative density differences and the detailed reproduction of the brain structures in the CT images are reduced by postmortem changes and fixation. As a result, these CT scans may produce images which are inconsistent with the diagnostic impression obtained after the examination of patients. The structures of these CT scans (Figs. 40a–d) are labelled and can be compared with the illustrations of the anatomical sections.

The brain mantle or pallium consists of the cerebral cortex and the white matter. The cerebral cortex is a 2 to 5 mm thick mantle of gray matter averaging 600 ml in males and 540 ml in females. This sex based volume difference is statistically significant. As a result of cytoarchitectonic, myeloarchitectonic, glio-architectonic, angioarchitectonic, chemoarchitectonic, and pigmentarchitectonic investigations, the cerebral cortex was divided into the allocortex and the isocortex. Mainly through comparative studies the allocortex was subdivided into the paleocortex and archeocortex bordered by a belt of peripaleocortex and periarcheocortex (289). The anterior perforated substance, the periamygdaloid cortex, and prepiriform cortex are part of the three- or four-layered paleocortex and form the cortical areas of the olfactory system (Chap. 4.7). The three-layered archeocortex consists of the dentate gyrus, hippocampus, and subiculum. These cortical formation and periarcheocortical areas in the parahippocampal gyrus, the subcallosal area, and the portions of the cingulate gyrus near the corpus callosum comprise the cortical portions of the limbic system

(Chap. 4.11). The periarcheocortex and peri-paleocortex are collectively known as mesocortex. The mesocortex is the transition to the six-layered isocortex. The isocortex corresponds to the neocortex refered to in comparative anatomy (287). Information gained from morphological, physiological, and clinical investigations indicates the following division of the isocortex:

● Primary cortical areas
● Secondary cortical areas
● Supplementary cortical areas.

The primary cortical areas have either afferent or efferent topical connections with the periphery. Basically, these are marked by point-to-point connections between the periphery and the cortex or vice versa. The anterolateral, medial lemniscus, and trigeminal systems project into the postcentral gyrus, into Brodmann's areas 3, 1, 2 (Figs. 12b.30, 13b.15, 14b.10, 15b.7, 16b.6, 17b.5, 18b.3). These cytoarchitectonic areas form three vertical bands arranged 3, 1, 2 from frontal to occipital in the postcentral gyrus (80). Their somatotopic order is described in Chapter 4.1. (sensory systems). The primary cortical area of the gustatory system is located in the parietal operculum and in an area on the edge of the insula (Chap. 4.2). The vestibular system has connections with the parietal cortex around the intraparietal sulcus. Located deep in the lateral sulcus in the transverse temporal gyri (Heschl), the auditory system has a large primary cortex in the temporal lobe (Figs. 12b.32 and 13b.21). Cytoarchitectonically, these areas correspond to Brodmann's areas 41 and 42. The visual primary cortical areas of both hemispheres have a volume of 12 ml. They can be recognized macroscopically by Vicq d'Azyr's band located in the occipital lobe in the upper and lower lips of the calcarine sulcus (Figs. 12b.44 and 53.17). There is a precise point-to-point projection from the retina to the visual cortex (Chap. 4.6).

The primary motor area or motor cortex is located in the frontal lobe and, for the most part, in and around the precentral gyrus (Figs. 12b.11, 13b.9, 14b.6, 15b.3, 16b.4, 17b.3, 18b.1). This location corresponds cytoarchitectonically to Brodmann's areas 4 and 6. Additional motor neurons arise from Brodmann's sensory areas 3, 1, 2 and their neighboring parietal areas (57, 106, 173). The somatotopic pattern of the motor cortex is described in Chapter 4.8.1 (pyramidal system).

During evolution of the neocortex, the secondary cortical areas developed between the primary areas in a mosaic pattern. This development is especially evident in primate brains. The secondary cortex is connected with other cortical areas or subcortical nuclei but not with motor neurons or sensory recep-

1 Frontal bone
2 Interhemispheric (lon-
    gitudinal cerebral) fis-
    sure
3 Frontal horn of lateral
    ventricle
4 Septum pellucidum
5 Cistern of lateral (Sylvian)
    fissure (insular cistern)
6 Third ventricle
7 Parietal bone
8 Lateral ventricle
9 Cistern of great cerebral
    vein (Galen)
10 Occipital bone
11 Choroid plexus
12 Splenium of corpus
    callosum
13 Collateral trigone of lateral
    ventricle
14 Cerebral falx
15 Central part of lateral
    ventricle
16 Semioval center

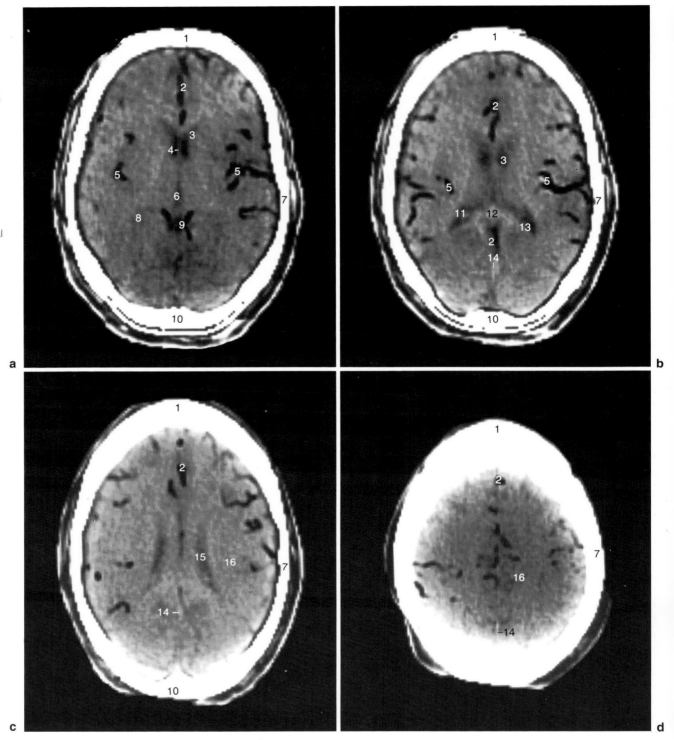

Fig. 40   Four CT images of the formalin-alcohol fixed head of a 44-year-old male. The corresponding levels of the individual slices can be found in Figures 1a, 2, 3, 4, 26.

Fig. 40a   CT image corresponds to the eighth slice (Figs. 12a, b). Frontal and occipital portions of the lateral ventricles are shown. The third ventricle can be recognized. The insular cistern, frontal interhemispheric fissure, and cistern of the great cerebral vein (Galen) are illustrated.

Fig. 40b   CT image corresponds to the ninth slice. The lateral ventricles with the frontal horns and collateral trigone are shown. The frontal and occipital interhemispheric fissure can be recognized.

Fig. 40c   CT image corresponds to the tenth slice. The central part of the lateral ventricle is shown.

Fig. 40d   CT image corresponds to the twelfth slice, which is in a supraventricular position.

tors in point-to-point relation. The secondary cortical areas have predominantly gnostic functions as "association areas". Included among the secondary areas are the motor language area located in the frontal operculum and the sensory language area located between the primary auditory area and the angular gyrus (Chap. 4.10).

The supplementary areas lie at the border between the primary cortex and phylogenetically older regions of the brain:

● The supplementary sensory area lies on the lateral surface of each hemisphere between the primary sensory cortex and insula (262).
● The supplementary auditory area is located on the lateral surface of the hemisphere between the primary auditory cortex and insula.
● The supplementary visual area lies on the medial surface of the hemisphere between the visual cortex and periarcheocortex (262).
● The supplementary motor area stretches on the medial surface of each hemisphere between Brodmann's area 4 and the paralimbic transitional cortex of the isocortex or proisocortex (28, 221).

The topical arrangement of the supplementary areas with the periphery is less developed than that of the primary areas. Nevertheless, a supplementary area can partially compensate the loss of the corresponding primary area.

The white matter underlying the cerebral cortex is formed by the many fibers of the various pathways that connect the cortical areas with each other or with other regions of the CNS. These connecting pathways include:

● Association fibers
● Commissural fibers
● Projection fibers.

The association (intrahemispheric) fibers are either short or long axonal projections that interconnect the cortical areas of one cerebral hemisphere. The short arcuate fibers lie directly beneath the cerebral cortex and appear as small connecting arches between adjacent gyri. The long association fibers interconnect the gyri of the individual cerebral lobes. The cingulum (Fig. 14b.9) is a fiber bundle located in the white matter of the cingulate gyrus. It arches around the corpus callosum from the frontal lobe to the temporal lobe.

The commissural (interhemispheric) fibers interconnect the corresponding cortical areas of the two hemispheres. The anterior commissure lies within the seventh section and is seen in the median view of the brain (Fig. 3.14). It connects the paleocortex (olfactory cortex) of one hemisphere with its counterpart in the contralateral hemisphere (Chap. 4.7).

In addition, the anterior commissure contains fibers that connect small neocortical areas of the frontal and temporal lobes with their counterparts. The corpus callosum is a large transverse connection between both sides of the neocortex. The divisions of the corpus callosum, the genu, trunk, and splenium, are depicted from frontal to occipital in the median view of the brain (Figs. 3.8, 3.5, 3.11).

The parallel canthomeatal illustrations show the genu of the corpus callosum (Figs. 11b.6 and 12b.6), a portion of the body (Fig. 13b.8), and the splenium (Fig. 13b.23). Two groups of U-shaped fibers emerge from the corpus. The frontal forceps (minor) (Fig. 13b.6) passes from the genu into the frontal lobes. The occipital forceps (major) (Fig. 13b.24) extends from the splenium into the occipital and temporal lobes.

The posterior commissure (Fig. 3.18) is not a commissural fiber bundle of the telencephalon. It connects nuclear areas in the tegmentum of the midbrain.

The projection fibers form afferent and efferent connections between the cerebral cortex and subcortical centers of the brain and spinal cord. The projection fibers of the telencephalon include the terminal fibers of the sensory (Chap. 4.1), gustatory (Chap. 4.2), vestibular (Chap. 4.4), auditory (Chap. 4.5), visual (Chap. 4.6), and olfactory (Chap. 4.7) systems. They also include the initial parts of pyramidal and oculomotor pathways (Chap. 4.8). The limbic system has many synaptic contacts via projection fibers with the diencephalon (Chap. 4.11). Portions of the monoaminergic system are also connected through fine projection fibers with the telencephalon (Chap. 4.12).

During evolution, the neencephalic projection fibers formed a crown of radiating fibers called the corona radiata (Fig. 13b.16). These projection fibers form the internal capsule. Lying in the diencephalic-telencephalic area, the internal capsule appears in the parallel canthomeatal planes as a fan-shaped band of fibers bent outward to form two limbs. The tip of the obtuse angle between these two limbs points in a medial direction. The internal capsule forms the medial border of the lentiform nucleus, a collective term for the globus pallidus and putamen. The internal capsule can be divided into an anterior limb, a genu, and a posterior limb. The anterior limb lies between the head of the caudate nucleus and the lentiform nucleus. The genu of the internal capsule lies between the anterior and posterior limbs at the level of the interventricular foramen (Monro). The posterior limb is located between the thalamus and the lentiform nucleus (Figs. 11b.17, 11b.18, 11b.19, 12b.7, 12b.19, 12b.20). The efferent projection fibers project into the genu and the adjacent portion of the posterior limb. The auditory and visual radiations are located in the retrolentiform part

(Chaps. 4.5 and 4.6). The projection fibers from the thalamus branch off in fan-shaped bundles that extend into the anterior and posterior limbs. A small number of the projection fibers forms the external capsule (Figs. 11b.12 and 12b.16), which is located between the putamen and claustrum. The fibers from the internal and external capsules converge in the cerebral peduncle of the midbrain (Fig. 10b.28). Projection fibers of the hippocampal formation project via the fimbria of the hippocampus and the fornix mainly to the hypothalamus (Figs. 12b.36, 12b.21, 11b.21, 13b.19).

The semioval center is the white matter of the telencephalon above the corpus callosum (Figs. 14b.14, 15b.8, 16b.7). In cross-sectional images, the white matter of one hemisphere above the corpus callosum appears semioval in shape. This semioval center consists of association, commissural, and projection fibers.

Depending on their relationship to neurofunctional systems in the individual lobes, telencephalic lesions will cause characteristic clinical symptoms enabling a preliminary topical diagnosis. A lesion in the motor cortex of the frontal lobe may take the form of an at least initially patterned convulsion (Jacksonian motor seizure). This begins with a tonic contraction of the fingers of one hand, one side of the face, or one foot and spreads to other muscles on the same side of the body. A severe acute lesion of the primary motor cortex produces a contralateral flaccid hemiplegia without significant spasticity. Only later may the reflexes be accentuated. Fine voluntary movements involving the distal muscles of the extremities will remain impaired. Lesions of the premotor cortex lead to a slowing of movements. Widespread injuries cause apraxia. Defects in the frontal operculum of the language-dominant hemisphere lead to motor aphasia. Injuries involving the base of the middle frontal gyrus may result in paralysis of the conjugate movement of the eyes; generally, the eyes will drift toward the side of the focus. Extensive lesions of the frontal lobe cause motor retardation or even akinesia. Furthermore, frontal lesions frequently elicit mental changes usually in the form of apathy or lack of initiative and emotional impairment. The close topographical relation of the frontal lobe and the olfactory bulb and tract explains the appearance of anosmia following pathological changes in the area of the anterior cranial fossa.

Parietal lesions in the postcentral gyrus lead to contralateral disturbances of peripheral sensitivity and spatial orientation. The perception of vibration and pain is seldom impaired. Abnormal stimulation of the parietal lobe may result in a sensory Jacksonian seizure. Characteristic symptoms for a parietal lobe syndrome are altered spatial and body orientation usually affecting the contralateral side; though very seldom, this may occur bilaterally.

In such cases, patients often forget activities such as putting a sock on the contralateral foot (dressing apraxia). Furthermore, spatial orientation may be impaired. Adolescents may develop muscle atrophy and skeletal hemiatrophy. An injury of the lower part of the parietal cortex in the hemisphere dominant for language causes alexia (74).

Lesions of the occipital lobe are marked by impairments of the contralateral visual field. Stimulation of the occipital lobe causes photopsia. Visual hallucinations arise with transient ischemia of the occipital pole and are frequently observed in connection with migraines (219). A complete bilateral loss of the visual cortex leads to cortical blindness.

Bilateral lesions of the transverse temporal gyri (Heschl) cause cortical deafness. Unilateral lesions, however, may remain clinically unnoticed. Pathology in the superior temporal gyrus leads to Wernicke's aphasia (86). Bilateral lesions of the hippocampal formation lead to memory and learning impairments or even to a severe amnestic syndrome. Injuries in the posterior region of the temporal lobe may cause homonymous hemianopsia or superior quadrantanopsia.

The commissural fibers of the corpus callosum serve the transmission of information from one hemisphere to the other. Interruption of the corpus callosum leads to a "disconnection effect". Lesions of the rostral portion of the corpus callosum produce an unilateral ataxia. Furthermore, tumors in this region may cause the patient to become apathetic. A severe loss of drive may result in mutism. Interruption of the trunk of the corpus callosum leads to a "tactile aphasia" (74). A patient with this lesion cannot name familiar objects held in the left hand (with eyes closed), although he indicates by gestures that he has identified them. Interruption of the splenium of the corpus callosum causes impairment of the patient's verbal articulation of experiences perceived in reading material in the right half of the visual field, but material in the left half would be meaningless.

4 Neurofunctional Systems

Neurofunctional systems are populations of neurons that process and transfer either specific afferent or efferent signals. Our description is restricted to those systems that may easily be tested clinically and that appear to be of diagnostic significance. In the case of the monoaminergic systems, however, an exception will be made. The latter systems are of importance in understanding neurobiochemical and neuropharmacological relationships. It is likely that in the future centers of neurobiochemical metabolism will be functionally analyzed using positron emission tomography (Chap. 2.2) and magnetic resonance imaging (Chap. 2.4). We believe, therefore, that a short description of the monoaminergic systems (Chap. 4.12) is necessary.

The successful description of pathways in the human nervous system is a synopsis of findings from neurohistological, neurophysiological, neuropathological, neurosurgical, neurological, animal experimental, and ontogenetic investigations. Modern tracing methods, e.g., horseradish peroxidase, can be used to detect neural connections in experimental animals only. As a result of neurosurgical stimulation tests conducted by Fritsch and Hitzig (78), the somatotopic organization of the pyramidal system in the human precentral gyrus has been known since 1870 and has been confirmed repeatedly (75, 206, 220). According to such clinical findings, the border between the motor innervation of the trunk and that of the head or, more specifically, the border between the corticospinal and corticonuclear areas lies in the precentral gyrus, approximately equidistant from the superior margin and the lateral sulcus (Sylvian fissure). Neurohistological findings indicate a gradual decrease in size of the giant cells (Betz) in area 4 as they extend from the superior margin to the lateral sulcus. To date there are no precise histological methods for localizing the point-to-point connections between the individual cortical nerve cells and the lower motor neurons suitable for human beings. Our illustrations, therefore, are based on a synopsis of contemporary knowledge gained from several fields of research concerning the probable topography of human neurofunctional systems.

In the prenatal phase, the neurofunctional systems are not fully developed, and the populations of embryonic nerve cells possess great plasticity (295). The younger the brain, the greater is the potential for compensation in case of a lesion. For example, if a cerebellum fails to form for genetic or environmental reasons, a different neuron population may almost totally take over its function. Cases of inborn cerebellar hypoplasia have been described, yet no cerebellar symptoms were observed during the entire lifetime. Similar observations have been made in cases of inborn aplasia of the corpus callosum (303). It is known that the infant brain can compensate for neurofunctional deficiencies much better than the adult brain, even though postnatal regeneration of nerve cells in the human brain is unlikely. A probable explanation for this compensation potential of neurofunctional deficiencies in infants would be the formation of new synaptic connections between already existing neurons. It has been shown in mammals that more nerve cells are formed prenatally and developed perinatally than actually function in postnatal life (31, 329). It is likely that infants initially possess a reserve of nerve cells that degenerate in the first two years of life. Not all prenatal and perinatal lesions can be compensated for and, as a result, some perinatal lesions may cause serious functional disorders. Blindness resulting from a bilateral occipital cortex defect is an example.

Even in adults, some lesions of cortical neurons, such as those of the language regions, can be compensated for. This is due to the existence of a cortical "reserve" of nerve cells, which results either from the lateralization of the hemispheres (Chap. 4.10) or the presence of supplementary regions (Chap. 3.6.5).

The positions of the neurofunctional systems in the various sectioning planes are presented in caudocranial order (Figs. 42–64). These serial illustrations are reproduced on the same scale as the CT scans. Individual areas have not been enlarged, as computed tomography does not possess a sufficient geometric resolution to image microscopic structures.

The difficulties inherent in transferring neuroanatomical findings from the cadaver to the corresponding in vivo situation are reviewed critically in Chapter 1.2. This problem must be taken into consideration in the analysis of the neurofunctional systems. Furthermore, individual variations of each neurofunctional system require additional investigation and clarification.

In spite of these limitations, hemianopsia, ataxia, aphasia, and many other lesions are diagnosed daily in clinical practice and are correlated with the probable region of the defect. Our illustrations of the main neurofunctional pathways drawn in the parallel canthomeatal planes should serve as an aid to diagnosis. We are convinced that the present knowledge of human neurofunctional pathways can be expanded by a scientific evaluation of the correlations observed between clinical, CT, and MR findings.

4.1 General Sensory Systems

4.1.1 Anterolateral System
(Figs. 41 and 42)

The anterolateral system receives its input from the pain, cold, warm, and mechanical receptors located in the legs, trunk, arms, and neck. The first sensory neurons have their pseudounipolar cell bodies in the spinal ganglia and terminate centrally in the marginal cells and cells of the nucleus proprius of the dorsal horn of the spinal cord. From there, the second neurons extend cranially as the anterior and lateral spinothalamic tracts and as spinoreticular tract. The spinothalamic tracts cross in the white commissure of the spinal cord and ascend contralaterally in the anterolateral funiculus. The spinoreticular tract extends (mainly ipsilaterally) as a polysynaptic pathway to the medial reticular formation of the brain stem and ascends further to the intralaminar nuclei of the thalamus. These thalamic neurons project widely throughout the cerebral cortex.

The spinothalamic tract extends alongside the reticular formation in the medulla oblongata and pons. In the pons-midbrain region it joins the medial lemniscus. Here an isolated lesion of only one pathway is unlikely. The spinothalamic tract terminates in the ventral posterolateral nucleus of the thalamus. From there the axons of the third neurons extend as thalamocortical fibers through the posterior limb of the internal capsule to the postcentral gyrus. Located in the postcentral gyrus is the sensory projection field (Brodmann's areas 3, 1, 2). In this narrow cortical area the somatosensory areas are organized somatotopically. The projection fields for the contralateral leg are localized on the superior margin. On the convex brain curvature, the areas for the trunk, arm, and neck of the opposite side extend toward the lateral sulcus. The axons of the third neurons pass also to the supplementary sensory area located in the parietal operculum near the insula. Interruption of the spinothalamic tract results in pain and temperature perception disorders (137, 146).

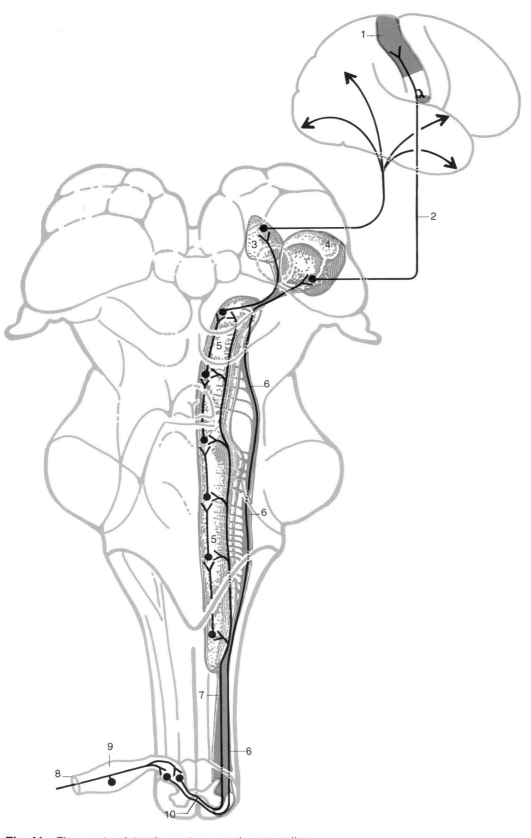

1 Postcentral gyrus
2 Thalamocortical fibers
3 Intralaminar nuclei of
   thalamus
4 Ventral posterolateral
   nucleus of thalamus
5 Medial reticular formation
6 Anterior and lateral
   spinothalamic tracts
7 Spinoreticular tract
8 Dorsal root of spinal nerve
9 Spinal ganglion
10 White commissure of
   spinal cord

Fig. 41 The anterolateral system and ascending reticular system in the spinal cord, medulla oblongata, pons, mesencephalon, and diencephalon as seen from a dorsal aspect and in the cerebrum as seen from a lateral aspect. According to (206).

1 Anterior and lateral
  spinothalamic tracts

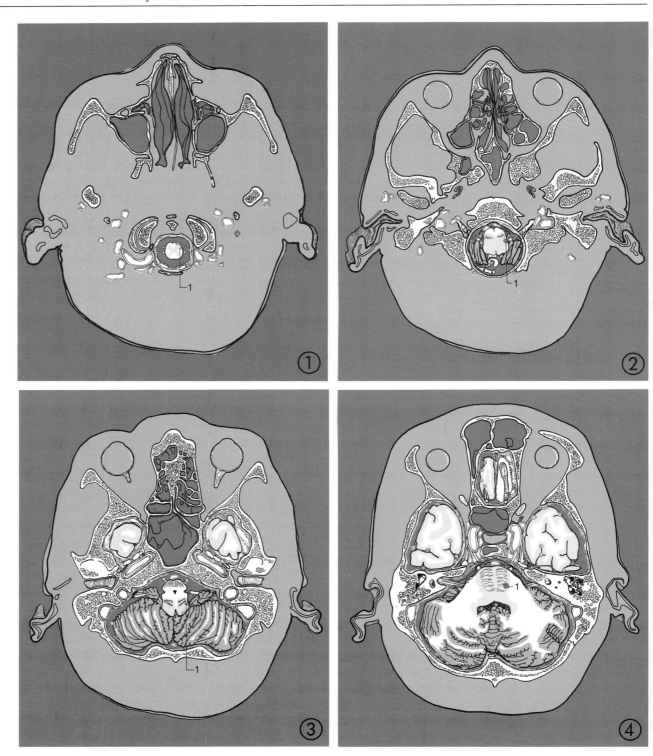

Fig. 42 Serial illustrations of the anterolateral system.
The encircled number indicates the number of the
respective slice (see Figs. 1a, 2, 3, 4).

1 Anterior and lateral
  spinothalamic tracts
2 Ventral posterolateral
  nucleus of thalamus
3 Thalamocortical fibers

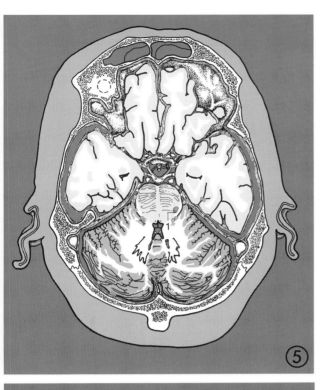

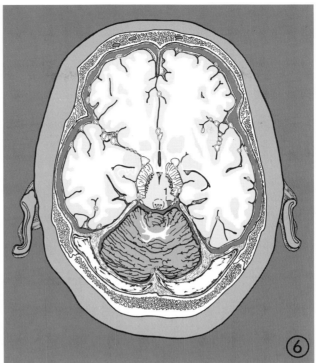

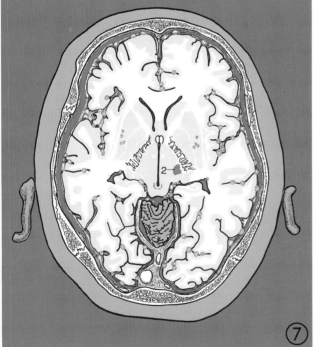

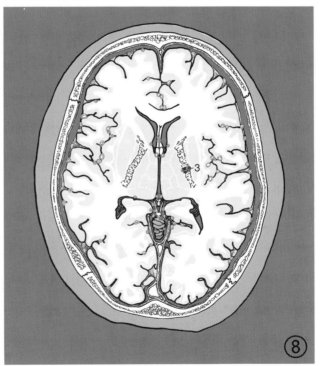

3 Thalamocortical fibers
4 Postcentral gyrus

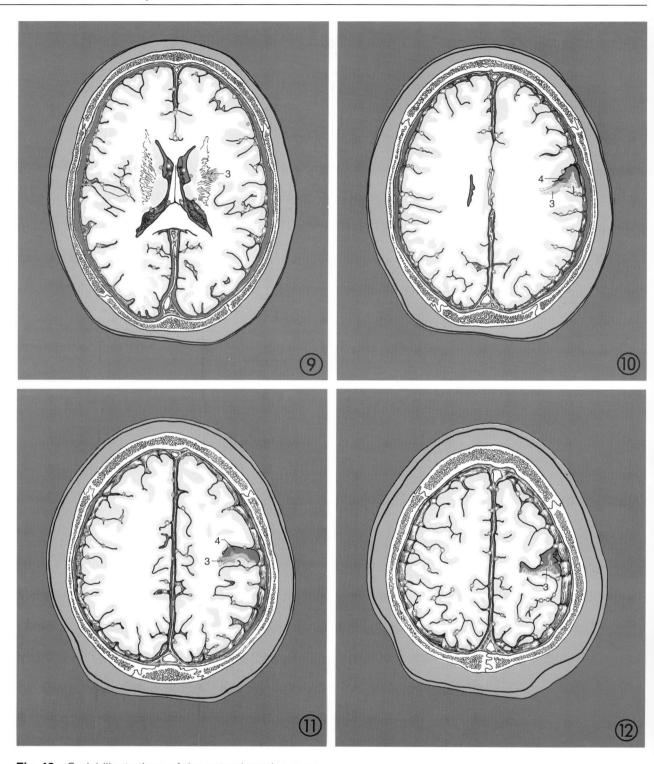

Fig. 42 Serial illustrations of the anterolateral system. The encircled number indicates the number of the respective slice (see Figs. 1a, 2, 3, 4).

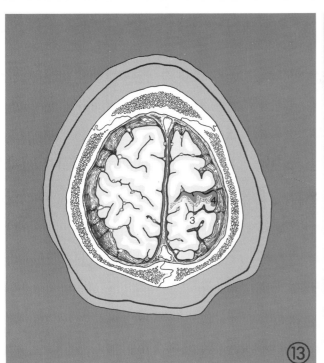

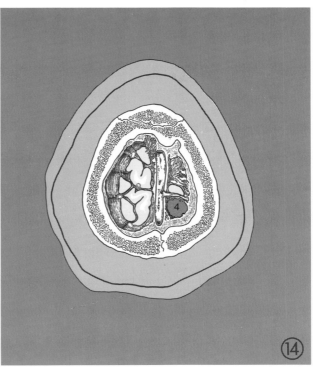

4.1.2 Medial Lemniscus System

(Figs. 43 and 44)

The receptors of the medial lemniscus system (dorsal column-lemniscal pathway (74, 140)) are the mechanical receptors in the skin, muscle spindles, tendon organs, and the proprioceptive stimulus transducers in the legs, trunk, arms, and neck. The cell bodies of the first neurons are located in the spinal ganglia. The axons of the pseudounipolar nerve cells enter the posterior funiculus of the spinal cord and are organized somatotopically; that is, the pathways from the individual dermatomes and myotomes are organized in layers. Axons from the caudal half of the body unite in the gracile fasciculus (medial spinobulbar tract) and those from the cranial half form the cuneate fasciculus (lateral spinobulbar tract).

In the medulla oblongata, the two fasciculi terminate in the gracile nucleus (Goll) and the cuneate nucleus (Burdach). From these nuclei, axons cross to the opposite side and ascend as the medial lemniscus. In a cross section through the medulla oblongata the two medial lemnisci appear as two fiber bundles that are in contact with each other in the median plane. In the pons, the medial lemniscus lies dorsal to the pontocerebellar pathways. In the midbrain, it occupies the lateral region of the tegmentum. It terminates in the ventral posterolateral nucleus of the thalamus. From this nucleus, the third neurons project as thalamocortical fibers through the posterior limb of the internal capsule to the postcentral gyrus and terminate in the sensory cortex (Brod-

mann's areas 3, 1, 2). This cortical area of the medial lemniscus system is somatotopically organized. The projection fields for the contralateral leg are localized on the superior margin. The areas for the trunk, arm and neck of the opposite side are located on the convex brain curvature.

An interruption of the medial lemniscus system leads to an impairment of proprioceptive perception (vibration and position senses) and of exteroceptive perception (disturbances of two-point discrimination). The perception of pain and temperature remains unaffected.

1 Postcentral gyrus
2 Thalamocortical fibers
3 Ventral posterolateral
 nucleus of thalamus
4 Medial lemniscus
5 Internal arcuate fibers
6 Cuneate nucleus
 (Burdach)
7 Gracile nucleus (Goll)
8 Cuneate fasciculus
 (Burdach) (lateral
 spinobulbar tract)
9 Gracile fasciculus (Goll)
 (medial spinobulbar tract)
10 Dorsal root of spinal nerve
11 Spinal ganglion

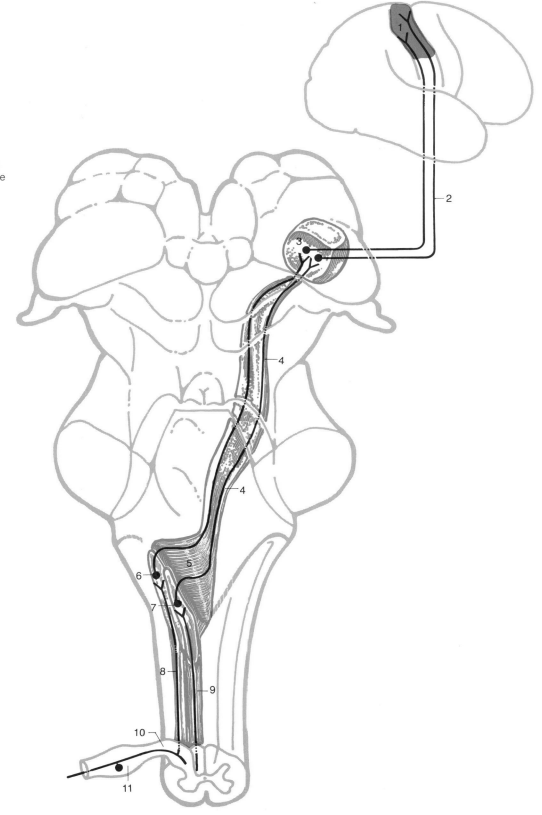

Fig. 43 The medial lemniscus system in the spinal cord, brain stem, and ciencephalon (dorsal view), and in the cerebrum (lateral view). According to (206).

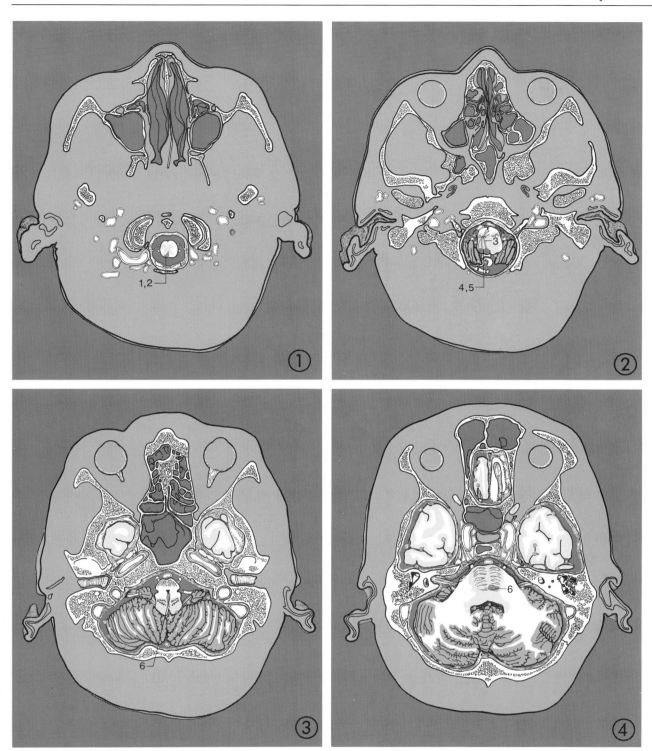

1 Cuneate fasciculus
  (Burdach) (lateral
  spinobulbar tract)
2 Gracile fasciculus (Goll)
  (medial spinobulbar tract)
3 Internal arcuate fibers
4 Cuneate nucleus (Burdach)
5 Gracile nucleus (Goll)
6 Medial lemniscus

Fig. 44 Serial illustrations of the medial lemniscus system. The encircled number indicates the number of the respective slice (see Figs. 1a, 2, 3, 4).

6 Medial lemniscus
7 Ventral posterolateral
  nucleus of thalamus
8 Thalamocortical fibers

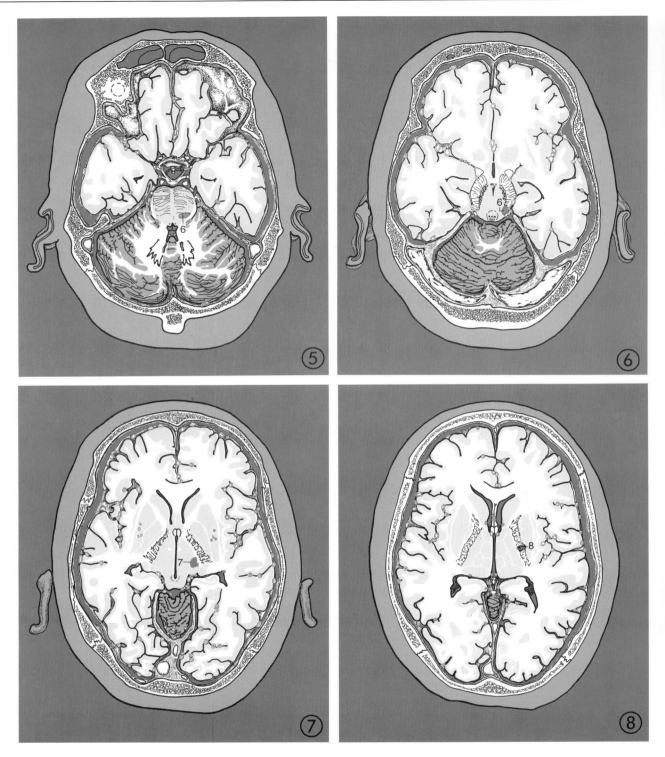

Fig. 44 Serial illustrations of the medial lemniscus system. The encircled number indicates the number of the respective slice (see Figs. 1a, 2, 3, 4).

8 Thalamocortical fibers
9 Postcentral gyrus

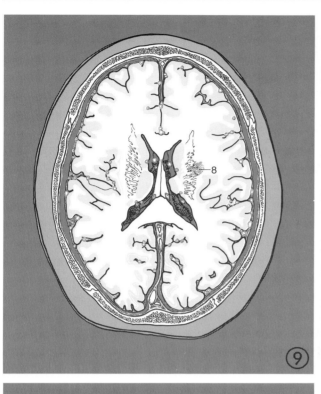

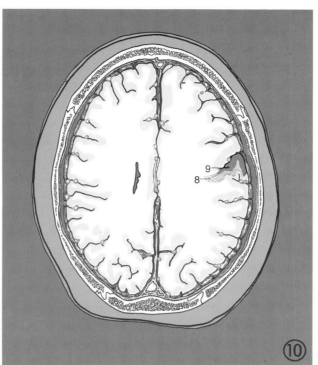

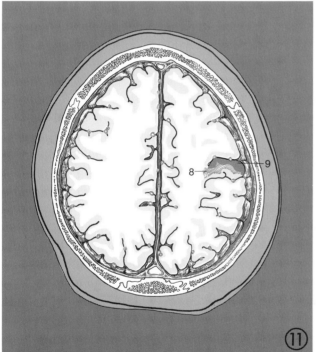

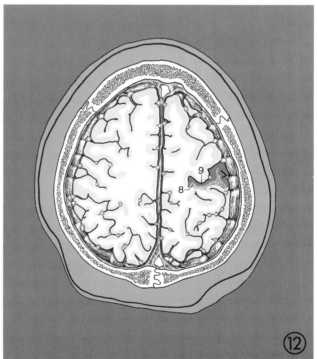

8 Thalamocortical fibers
9 Postcentral gyrus

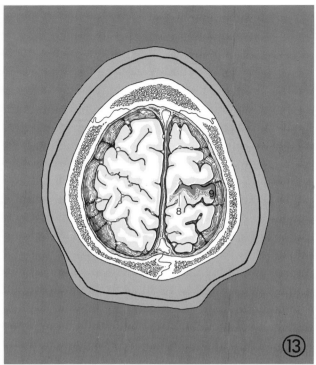

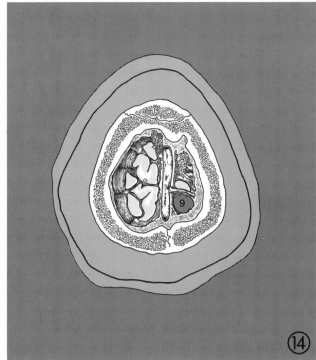

Fig. 44

4.1.3 Trigeminal System

(Figs. 36, 45, 46)

The pain, cold, and warm receptors of the facial skin, as well as those of the mucous membranes of the nose with its paranasal sinuses, the oral cavity, and the teeth transmit their signals via branches of the trigeminal nerve to the pseudounipolar nerve cells of the trigeminal (Gasserian) ganglion. The central projections of the trigeminal ganglion extend via the sensory root of the trigeminal nerve to the spinal nucleus of the trigeminal nerve. This nucleus is located lateral in the medulla oblongata and extends into the upper cervical spinal cord. It corresponds to the marginal cells and cells of the nucleus proprius of the posterior horn of the spinal cord, which also transmit pain, cold, and warm signals. Arising from the spinal trigeminal nucleus, the next neurons cross in the medulla oblongata, ascend as the trigeminothalamic tract, and synapses in the ventral posteromedial nucleus of the thalamus. The axons of the third neurons reach the postcentral gyrus and the supplementary sensory area (Chap. 4.1.1). The primary area for these pathways is located at the base of the postcentral gyrus close to the lateral sulcus.

The mechanoreceptors of the facial skin, eyes, and nasal and oral cavities transmit their information via branches of the trigeminal nerve to the pseudounipolar nerve cells of the trigeminal ganglion. The central axons of the trigeminal ganglion extend as the sensory root (portio major) of the trigeminal nerve to the main sensory (pontine) nucleus of the trigeminal nerve. This nucleus is located in the pons. From the main sensory nucleus the second neurons cross over to the opposite side and extend in the trigeminal lemniscus alongside the medial lemniscus, to the ventral posteromedial nucleus of the thalamus. Thalamocortical fibers reach the postcentral gyrus. Both pathways transmit exteroceptive and proprioceptive sensory signals with the exception of pain and temperature modalities (53). In primates, uncrossed fibers extending to the thalamus have been described (282).

The muscle spindle afferents of the masticatory muscles pass through pseudounipolar nerve cells which are not located in the trigeminal ganglion. These nerve fibers reach their pseudounipolar nerve cells in the mesencephalic nucleus of the trigeminal nerve located beside the central gray of the midbrain. Their central axons form a collateral to the motor nucleus of the trigeminal nerve. The masseter reflex can be triggered by means of this monosynaptic pathway.

4.1.4 Topography of Sensory Disorders

The separate courses of the anterolateral system and the medial lemniscus system in the medulla oblongata explain the appearance of a dissociated sensory disorder as a result of an isolated lesion of the anterolateral system in the medulla oblongata. Small vascular lesions in the anterolateral system cause a contralateral loss of pain and temperature sensation with preservation of tactile sensivity. With an additional lesion of the primary trigeminal neurons and/

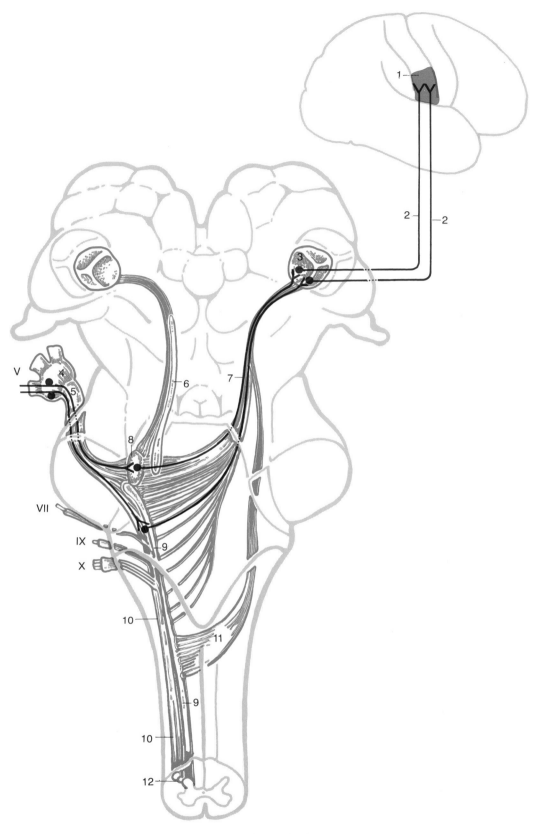

1 Postcentral gyrus
2 Thalamocortical fibers
3 Ventral posteromedial nucleus of thalamus (nucleus ventrocaudalis internus (107))
4 Trigeminal (Gasserian) ganglion
5 Sensory root of trigeminal nerve
6 Mesencephalic nucleus of trigeminal nerve
7 Trigeminal lemniscus
8 Main sensory (pontine) nucleus of trigeminal nerve
9 Spinal nucleus of trigeminal nerve
10 Spinal tract of trigeminal nerve
11 Lateral trigeminothalamic tract
12 Gelatinous substance (Rolando)

V   Trigeminal nerve
VII Facial nerve
IX   Glossopharyngeal nerve
X   Vagus nerve

Fig. 45 The trigeminal system in the spinal cord, brain stem, and diencephalon (dorsal view), and in the cerebrum (lateral view). Roman numerals indicate the cranial nerves. According to (206).

1 Spinal tract of trigeminal
  nerve
2 Spinal nucleus of trigeminal
  nerve
3 Lateral trigeminothalamic
  tract (within the slice)
4 Lateral trigeminothalamic
  tract
5 Trigeminal (Gasserian)
  ganglion
6 Main sensory (pontine)
  nucleus of trigeminal
  nerve

V   Trigeminal nerve
V/2   Maxillary nerve
V/3   Mandibular nerve

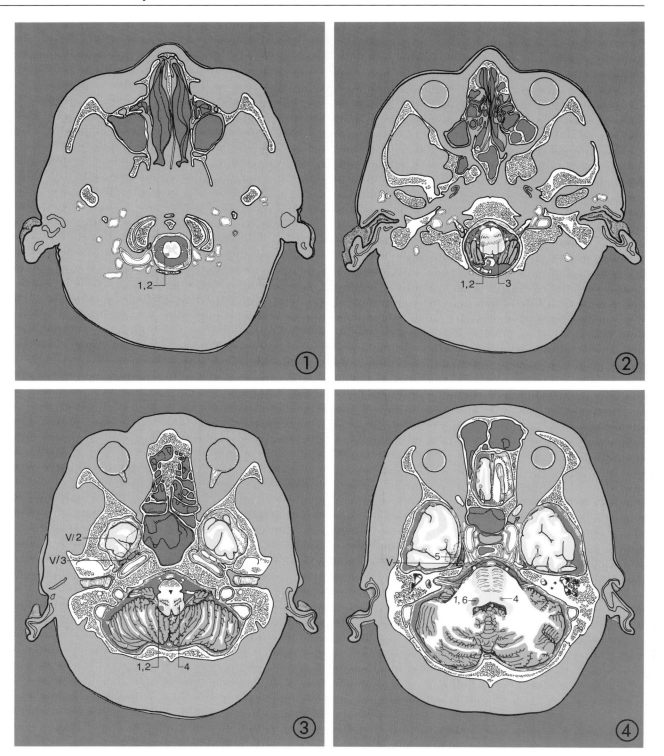

Fig. 46 Serial illustrations of the trigeminal system.
The encircled number indicates the number of the
respective slice (see Figs. 1a, 2, 3, 4).

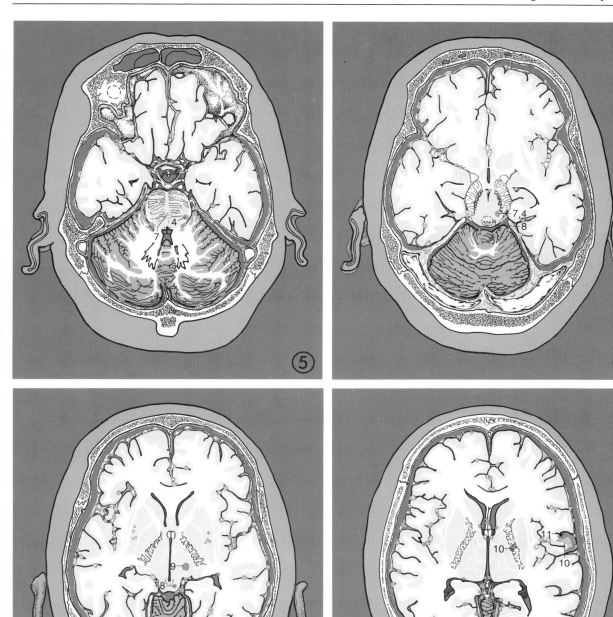

4 Lateral trigeminothalamic
  tract
7 Trigeminal lemniscus
8 Mesencephalic nucleus of
  trigeminal nerve
9 Ventral posteromedial
  nucleus of thalamus
10 Thalamocortical fibers
11 Postcentral gyrus

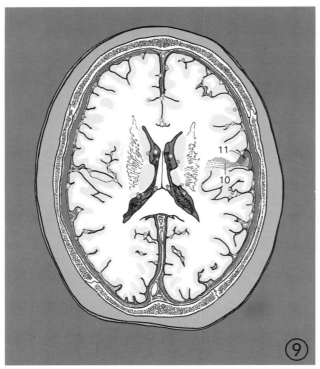

Fig. 46

or of the initial part of the secondary trigeminal neurons, ipsilateral sensory impairments will develop in the face. This produces a crossed impairment, such as that of the Wallenberg's syndrome, caused by lesions in the lateral medulla oblongata. A lesion of the medial lemniscus system impairs tactile discrimination, i.e., sensations of touch, position, and vibration. Lesions near the midline of the medulla oblongata may give rise to impairments on one or both sides of this sensory system. Due to the close proximity of both sensory systems further cranially, dissociated sensory disorders above the pons are rare. The same is true for the trigeminal system. Isolated pain and temperature sensory disorders arise only in connection with injuries of the upper cervical spinal cord and/or the medulla oblongata.

Foci in the posterior region of the internal capsule usually cause sensory disorders affecting the entire contralateral side of the body. This is due to the compact bundling of all sensory systems in this area. Increasing somatotopic fanning of the thalamocortical pathways in the semioval center, as they extend toward the sensory cortex, results in isolated sensory disorders of individual (contralateral) parts of the body. Such disorders include the entire range of sensory qualities.

4.2 Gustatory System (Figs. 47 and 48)

The facial, glossopharyngeal, and vagus nerves receive gustatory signals from the taste buds and free nerve endings and transmit these signals to the medulla oblongata. The cell bodies of the first neurons are located in the ganglia of the seventh (VII), ninth (IX), and tenth (X) cranial nerves: the geniculate ganglion and the superior and inferior ganglia of IX and X. The central axons of the pseudounipolar nerve cells terminate in the gustatory part of the solitary nucleus and in its rostral extension, the nucleus ovalis. The continuing pathway takes an ascending route similar to that of the trigeminal system close to the medial lemniscus and reaches the ventral posteromedial nucleus of the thalamus. The third neurons project from here to the opercular region of the parietal lobe and to an area on the edge of the insula (12, 40). Impairments of the sense of taste are predominantly accounted for by peripheral lesions of the taste buds or lesions of the seventh, ninth, and/or tenth cranial nerves.

4.3 Ascending Reticular System
(Fig. 41)

The reticular formation consists of a network of organized nerve cells in the medial tegmentum of the medulla oblongata, pons, and midbrain. The cranial nerve nuclei, several relay nuclei, and the descending pathways surround the reticular formation. The medial lemniscus system passes through it (232).

The reticular formation receives afferent signals from the spinal cord and from all sensory cranial nerves. These signals are relayed through the intralaminar thalamic nuclei via widespread projections to the cerebral cortex. Due to its polysynaptic conduction of impulses and extensive overlap, the reticular formation forms a nonspecific system of neurons extending between the receptors and the cortical nerve cells. In contrast to this nonspecific system, are the specific processing systems, with a point-to-point relay between the signal producing receptors and the nerve cells in the primary cortical areas. Examples of specific signal processing systems include the medial lemniscus system and the visual pathway. The ascending reticular system projects into numerous subcortical centers, such as the striatum, septum verum, and hypothalamus (27, 206). It should also be noted that the ascending reticular system is closely connected with the descending reticular system (33).

The complex relay arrangement of the reticular formation with its numerous connections to the motor systems, limbic system, and a great number of other systems explains the difficulty in analyzing isolated functional disorders. Lesions of the reticular system may result in either a disorder or a total loss of consciousness.

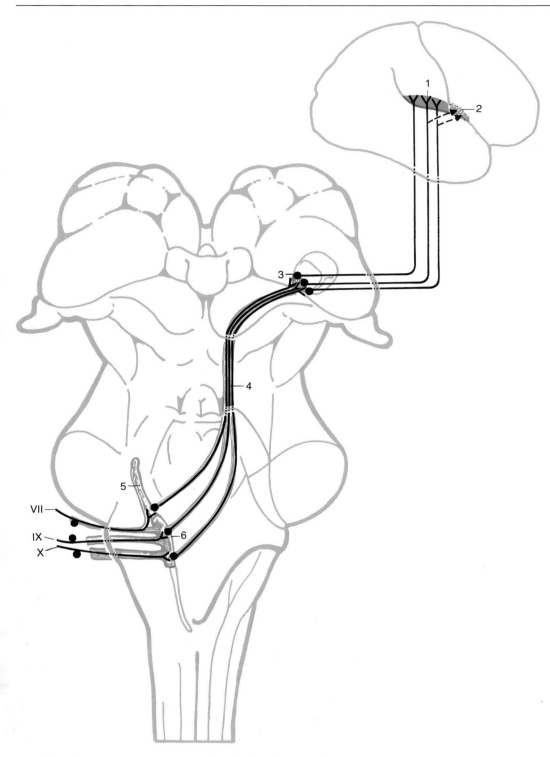

1 Parietal operculum
2 Gustatory cortical area near the margin of insula
3 Ventral posteromedial nucleus of thalamus
4 Gustatory fibers in dorsal trigeminothalamic tract
5 Nucleus ovalis
6 Pars gustatoria of solitary nucleus

Fig. 47 The gustatory system in the brain stem and diencephalon (dorsal view), and in the cerebrum (lateral view). Roman numerals indicate the facial, glossopharyngeal, and vagus nerves. According to (206).

1 Glossopharyngeal nerve and vagus nerve
2 Facial nerve and chorda tympani
3 Solitary nucleus (within the slice)
4 Gustatory fibers in dorsal trigeminothalamic tract

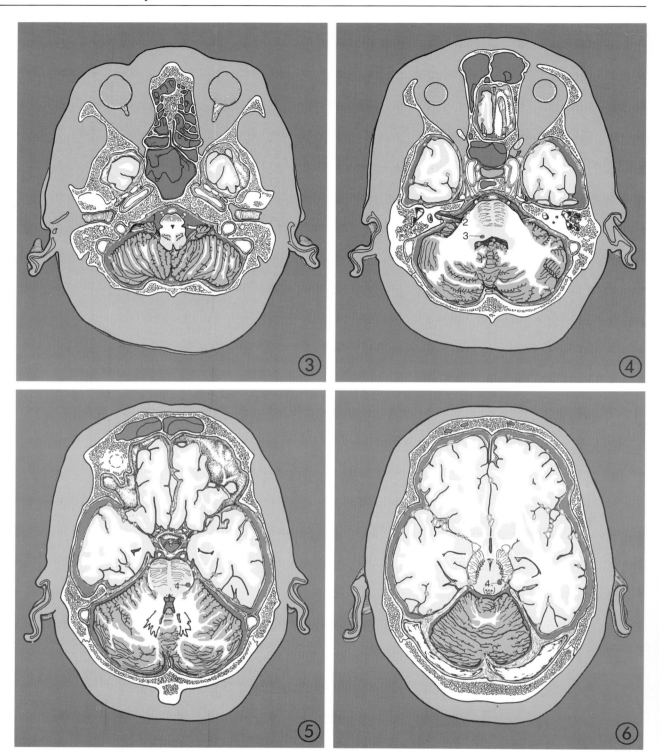

Fig. 48 Serial illustrations of the gustatory system. The encircled number indicates the number of the respective slice (see Figs. 1a, 2, 3, 4).

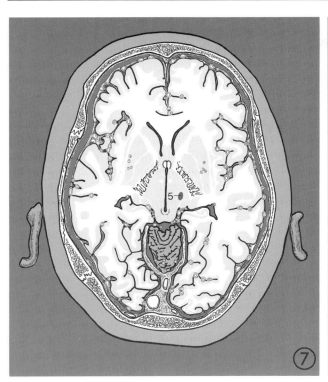

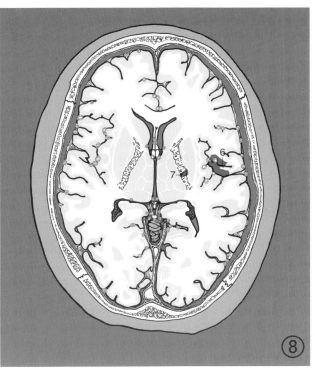

5 Ventral posteromedial
   nucleus of thalamus
6 Parietal operculum
7 Hypothetical fibers from
   thalamus to parietal operculum

4.4 Vestibular System (Figs. 49 and 50)

The receptors of the vestibular system are located in the semicircular ducts and in the saccule and utricle. The sensory cells of the semicircular ducts monitor angular acceleration of the head. The sensory cells in the saccule and utricle are covered by small calcium crystals embedded in a gelatinous layer and emit signals describing the effect of gravity on the body. In this way, information may be registered concerning linear acceleration in the earth's field of gravity. The signals of angular and linear acceleration are transmitted by the neurons of the vestibular system. The perikarya of the first vestibular neurons are located in the internal acoustic (auditory) meatus in the vestibular ganglion. The peripheral axons of these bipolar cells branch close to the sensory cells of the semicircular ducts as well as to those of the saccule and utricle. The central axons form the vestibular portion of the eighth cranial nerve, which enters the brain stem at the cerebellopontine angle. The fibers connected to the sensory cells of the semicircular ducts terminate primarily at the superior vestibular nucleus or extend directly to the flocculonodular lobe of the cerebellum. The fibers connected synaptically to the sensory cells in the saccule and utricle, extend to the medial and inferior vestibular nuclei. Only a few of the primary vestibular afferent nerves terminate in the large-celled lateral vestibular nucleus (Deiters).

The vestibular nuclei receive afferent signals from the spinal cord, reticular formation, and cerebellum. Efferent connections extend as the lateral vestibulospinal tract from the lateral vestibular nucleus to the spinal cord. The remaining vestibular nuclei send their fibers via the medial longitudinal fasciculus to the motor neurons of the neck and eye muscles. These pathways build a navigational system that compensates for external disturbances and stabilizes the position of the eyes and posture of the head. Each movement of the head is followed by oculomotor reflexes that maintain the position of an observed object on a fixed point on the retina. In this way, constant optical orientation in space is achieved.

In total, the vestibular system has numerous connections with the motor neurons of the eye, neck, trunk, arm, and leg muscles (vestibular reflexes).

There are few connecting pathways between the vestibular system and the cerebral cortex. They probably extend to the small contralateral ventral intermediate nucleus (107) of the thalamus and further to a parietal cortical area around the intraparietal sulcus (32, 77, 154).

Vestibular system deficiencies result in a lack of equilibrium. Acute vestibular lesions initially cause vertigo (a spinning sensation). Unilateral deficiencies of the vestibular system are compensated for after a period of several days or weeks, whereas bilateral lesions lead to a consistently unsteady gait (62, 196, 197). An involuntary, spontaneous, or reflex movement of both eyeballs is referred to as nystagmus. A nystagmus is characterized by both a slow and a rapid component. Peripheral disorders affect the receptors in the semicircular ducts and/or the first vestibular neuron. Central disorders influence the other neurons of the vestibular system. Gaze-dependent nystagmus is observed as a result of lesions in the cerebellum, the medulla oblongata, and mesencephalic oculomotor regions (39). Fixation nystagmus can be identified by the pendular movement of the eyes upon fixation and is a congenital disorder of the corticonuclear oculomotor system. Spontaneous nystagmus is one that can be observed as soon as visual fixation is eliminated by Frenzel's glasses. It is found in connection with both peripheral and central disorders. Because different lesions may cause similar forms of nystagmus, the classification of a nystagmus alone is not sufficient for an adequate topical diagnosis. A dissociated nystagmus, however, points to a midline lesion located in the area of the eye muscle nuclei in the brain stem especially in the medial longitudinal fasciculus at this level. With dissociated nystagmus, the abducted eye shows a significantly larger deflection of the eyeball. Rotatory and vertical nystagmus also indicate the presence of a central lesion.

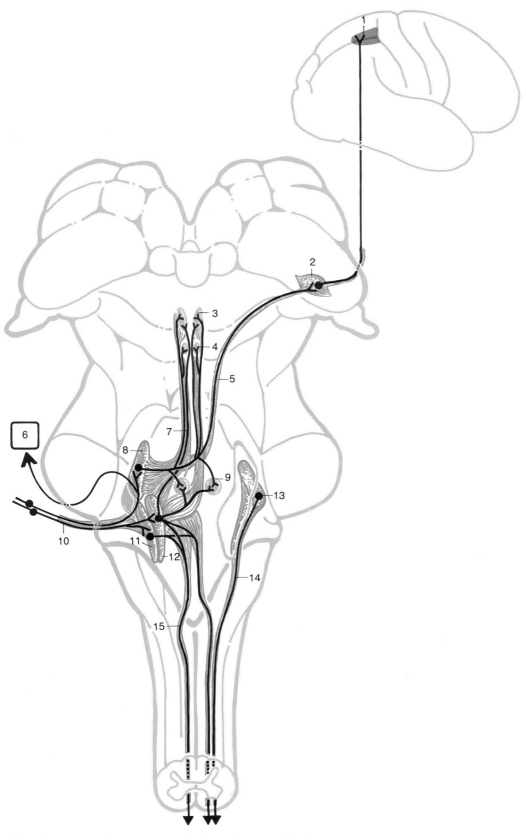

1 Vestibular cortical area in parietal lobe
2 Ventral intermediate nucleus of thalamus
3 Oculomotor nucleus
4 Trochlear nucleus
5 Vestibulothalamic tract
6 Cerebellum
7 Medial longitudinal fasciculus
8 Superior vestibular nucleus
9 Abducens nucleus
10 Vestibular part of vestibulocochlear nerve
11 Inferior vestibular nucleus
12 Medial vestibular nucleus
13 Lateral vestibular nucleus (Deiters)
14 Lateral vestibulospinal tract
15 Medial vestibulospinal tract

Fig. 49 The vestibular system in the spinal cord, brain stem, and diencephalon (dorsal view), and in the cerebrum (lateral view). According to (206).

1 Medial vestibulospinal tract
2 Lateral vestibulospinal tract
3 Vestibular part of
   vestibulocochlear nerve
4 Vestibular nuclei
5 Lateral vestibular nucleus
   (Deiters)

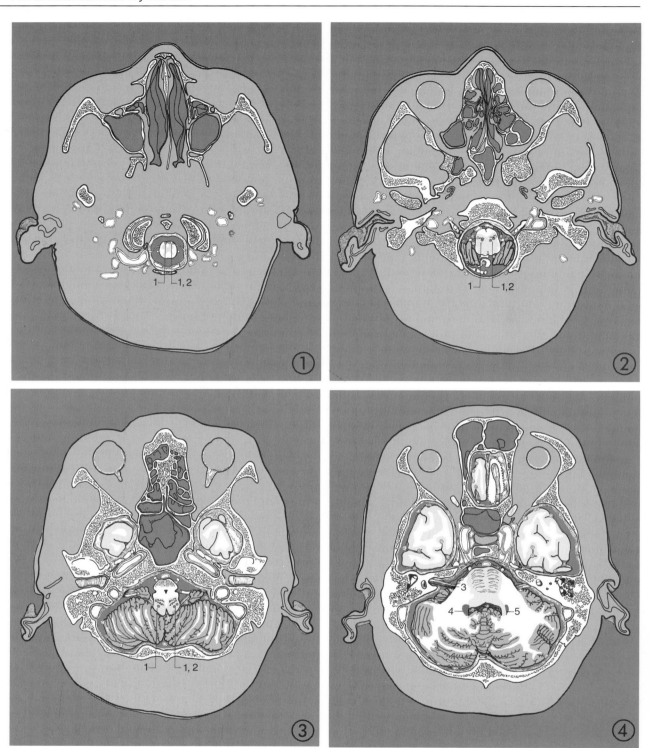

Fig. 50 Serial illustrations of the vestibular system. The encircled number indicates the number of the respective slice (see Figs. 1a, 2, 3, 4).

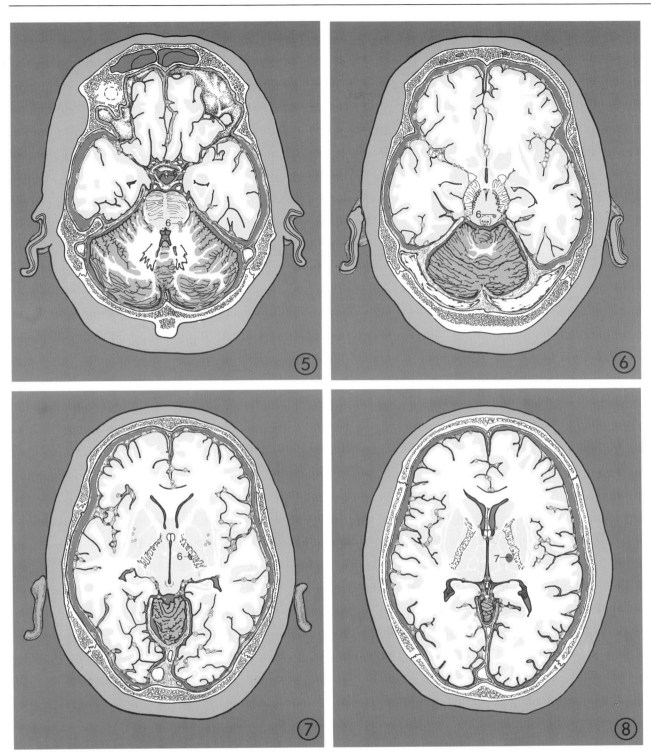

6 Vestibulothalamic tract
7 Ventral intermediate
  nucleus of thalamus
  (within the slice)

8 Hypothetical fibers from
  thalamus to parietal cortex
9 Vestibular cortical area in
  parietal lobe

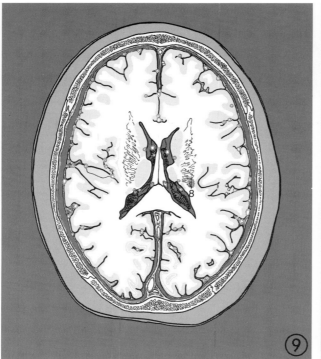

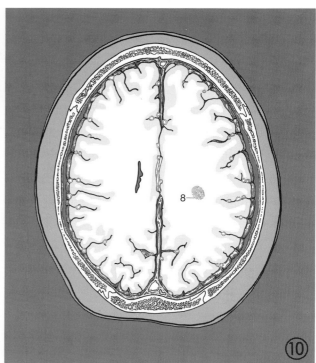

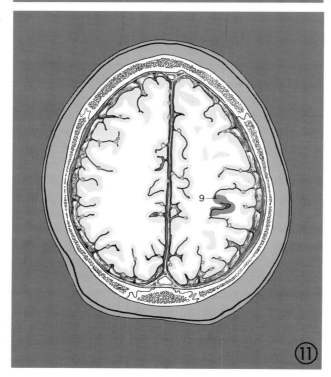

Fig. 50 Serial illustrations of the vestibular system.
The encircled number indicates the number of the
respective slice (see Figs. 1a, 2, 3, 4).

4.5 Auditory System (Figs. 51 and 52)

Sound waves reach the tympanic membrane through the external acoustic (auditory) meatus. The auditory ossicles mechanically amplify vibrations in the middle ear and send them toward the oval window. The resulting endolymphatic movements are perceived by the hair cells of the spiral organ (Corti) in the inner ear and are transmitted to the chain of neurons in the auditory system.

Anatomically speaking, retrocochlear hearing impairment is a lesion of this chain of neurons. The first neurons of this chain are formed in the cochlea by the bipolar nerve cells of the spiral ganglion. Their peripheral processes are connected with the base of the hair cells in the spiral organ (Corti). The central axons of the bipolar cells form the cochlear portion of the eighth cranial nerve. The axons emerge near the opening of the internal acoustic meatus from the petrous portion of the temporal bone and enter the medulla oblongata at the cerebellopontine angle. The central axons subsequently divide into two branches, one extending toward the dorsal cochlear nucleus and the other toward the ventral cochlear nucleus. The secondary auditory neurons originate in these two nuclei.

● The axons of the dorsal cochlear nucleus pass along the floor of the rhomboid fossa just beneath the medullary striae of the fourth ventricle. They cross over to the opposite side and run in the lateral lemniscus to the inferior colliculus. Along the way, an additional neuron may be interposed. The axons of the nerve cells of the inferior colliculus conduct the auditory signals by way of the brachium of the inferior colliculus to the medial geniculate body. The final neurons extend from the medial geniculate body through the auditory radiation to the primary auditory cortex (areas 41 and 42). The latter is located in the transverse temporal gyri (Heschl) on the floor of the lateral sulcus (101).

● The ventral auditory pathway in the trapezoid body extends from the ventral cochlear nucleus to the superior olivary nucleus and the nuclei of the trapezoid body, crossing to the opposite side to join the lateral lemniscus. Together these two pathways continue in the same manner as the dorsal part of the auditory pathway already described. A second portion of the ventral auditory pathway remains on the same side and extends ipsilaterally by way of the above mentioned subcortical centers to the primary auditory cortex of the cerebrum (areas 41 and 42). This bilateral construction of the auditory pathway probably plays a role in directional hearing.

Several of the nuclei mentioned are not merely relay nuclei but also reflex centers, through which the nuclei of the trapezoid body are connected with the motor nuclei of the fifth and seventh cranial nerves. In this manner, two reflex arcs are formed from the spiral organ (Corti) to the tensor tympani and stapedius muscles. As a reflex response to high intensity tones, the muscles contract and consequently dampen the transmission of sound waves from the tympanic membrane to the stapes. Loss of this reflex results in hyperacusis (painful sensitivity to loud sounds). Additional reflex pathways extend from the inferior colliculus to the superior colliculus. These pathways modulate reflexes associated with eye and head movements caused by auditory stimuli. Furthermore, the neurons of the reticular formation are interconnected with the ascending portion of the auditory pathway.

Originating in the superior olivary nucleus, an efferent pathway extends into the cochlea and terminates on the hair cells of the spiral organ (Corti) (olivocochlear bundle of Rasmussen). Experimentally, impulses arising in the auditory nerve can be suppressed by stimulation of this olivocochlear tract.

Clinically, middle ear, cochlear, and retrocochlear hearing impairments can be differentiated. Recognition of middle ear deafness involves a simple examination using a tuning fork. To distinguish a cochlear or retrocochlear hearing defect, neurophysiological tests such as the computerized Auditory Evoked Potentials (AEP) or Brainstem Electric Response Audiometry (BERA) are utilized. An X-ray examination of the petrous portion of the temporal bones, including X-ray tomography and high resolution computed tomography, is an additional step in the diagnosis of hearing impairments of uncertain origin. Furthermore, postinfusion computed tomography is of importance when examining patients with a suspected cerebellopontine angle tumor. In cases of cortical hearing impairment, CT is the most important diagnostic tool available since an EEG will provide diagnostic hints only. Paracusia and auditory hallucinations may be caused by temporal lobe disorders.

1 Transverse temporal gyri
   (Heschl)
2 Acoustic radiation
3 Medial geniculate body
4 Brachium of inferior
   colliculus
5 Inferior colliculus
6 Commissure of inferior
   colliculus
7 Lateral lemniscus
8 Nucleus of lateral
   lemniscus
9 Superior olivary nuclei
10 Cochlear part of
   vestibulocochlear
   nerve
11 Ventral cochlear nucleus
12 Trapezoid body
13 Nuclei of trapezoid body
14 Dorsal cochlear nucleus
15 Medullary striae of fourth
   ventricle

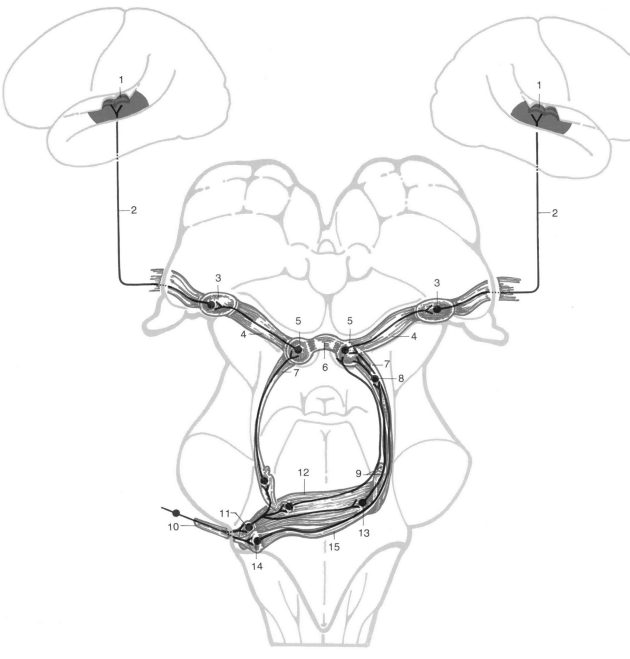

Fig. 51 The auditory system in the brain stem and diencephalon (dorsal view), and in the cerebrum (lateral view). According to (206).

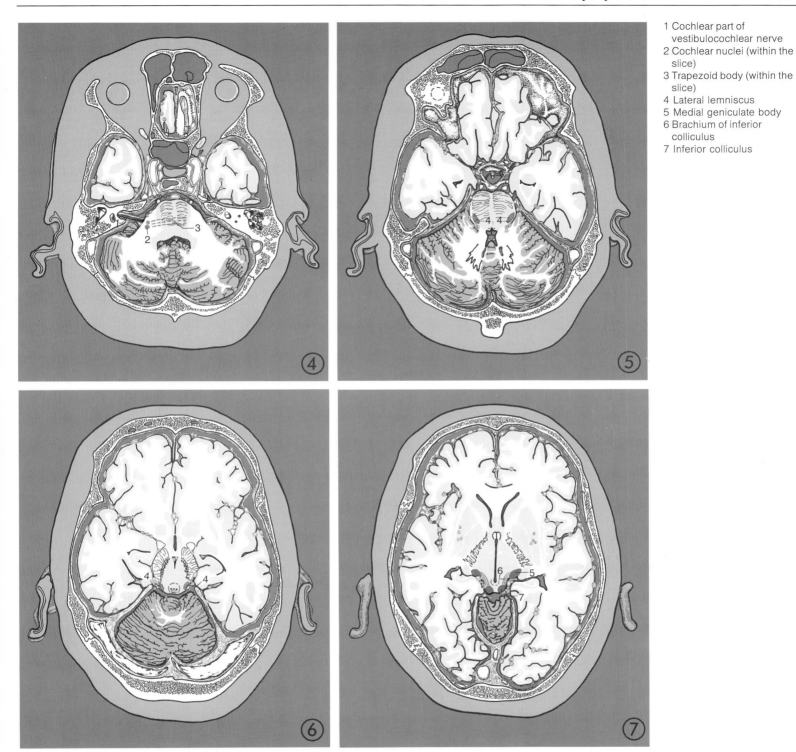

1 Cochlear part of
  vestibulocochlear nerve
2 Cochlear nuclei (within the
  slice)
3 Trapezoid body (within the
  slice)
4 Lateral lemniscus
5 Medial geniculate body
6 Brachium of inferior
  colliculus
7 Inferior colliculus

Fig. 52 Serial illustrations of the auditory system. The encircled number indicates the number of the respective slice (see Figs. 1a, 2, 3, 4).

8 Acoustic radiation
9 Transverse temporal gyri
   (Heschl)

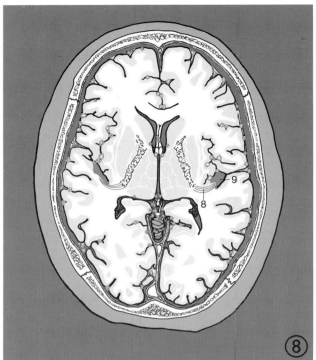

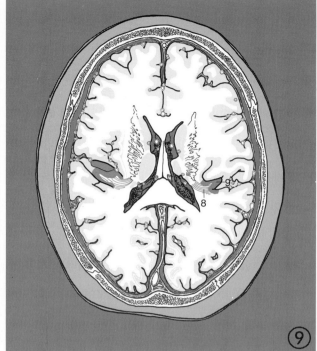

Fig. 52

4.6 Visual System (Figs. 53 and 54)

The photoreceptors of the visual system are located in the retina. Optical signals emitted from the rods and cones are transmitted through bipolar nerve cells to large multipolar ganglion cells. The axons of these ganglion cells extend along the inner layer of the retina and converge at the optic disk. These axons pass through the lamina cribrosa of the sclera and form the optic nerve. Within the orbit, the optic nerve measures 2.5 cm in length and has a slightly curved path to allow for free eye movements. The optic nerve crosses the canthomeatal plane at an acute angle and can, therefore, be seen in three of the 1 cm thick slices (Fig. 54.2). The optic nerve extends towards the optic chiasm through the optic canal, a bony channel approximately 5 mm in length (Fig. 54.3). As the eye moves laterally, the optic nerve is repositioned somewhat medially in the orbit (260). Within the orbit, the optic nerve is sheathed by the pia, arachnoid, and dura mater with a narrow subarachnoid space. In the optic canal, dura mater and bone have grown tightly together.

Caudal to the optic chiasm lie the sphenoid sinus and the sella turcica with the pituitary gland (hypophysis). The optic chiasm is located in front of the hypothalamus and medial to the internal carotid arteries.

Fibers from the nasal half of the retina only (temporal visual field) cross in the optic chiasm, while fibers from the temporal half of the retina (nasal visual field) remain on the same side. The crossed and uncrossed fibers form the optic tract which is approx-imately 4 cm long. This arches along the border between the diencephalon and telencephalon to the lateral geniculate body where most of the fibers terminate (Fig. 54.4).

About 10% of the optic tract fibers extend to the superior colliculi and pretectal areas. The reflexes of the intrinsic and extrinsic eye muscles are modulated via this portion of the optic nerve. A third group of fibers forms the extrageniculate pathway leading to the cerebral cortex (see below).

The visual pathway leaves the lateral geniculate body as the optic radiation (geniculocalcarine tract) and loops over the temporal horn of the lateral ventricle before turning medially toward the visual cortex around the calcarine sulcus (45, 46, 87). The cells of the medial half of the lateral geniculate body project into the upper portion of the visual cortex. This part of the optic radiation extends backward in a short loop from the internal capsule to the upper lip of the visual cortex. The other part of the optic radiation, which arises from the lateral half of the lateral geniculate body, extends initially in a large arc into the temporal lobe. From here it continues toward the lower lip of the visual cortex (Fig. 54.7) in a loop lateral to the temporal horn of the lateral ventricle. A lesion located in this lateral part of the optic radiation impairs perception in the upper quadrant of the visual field (110).

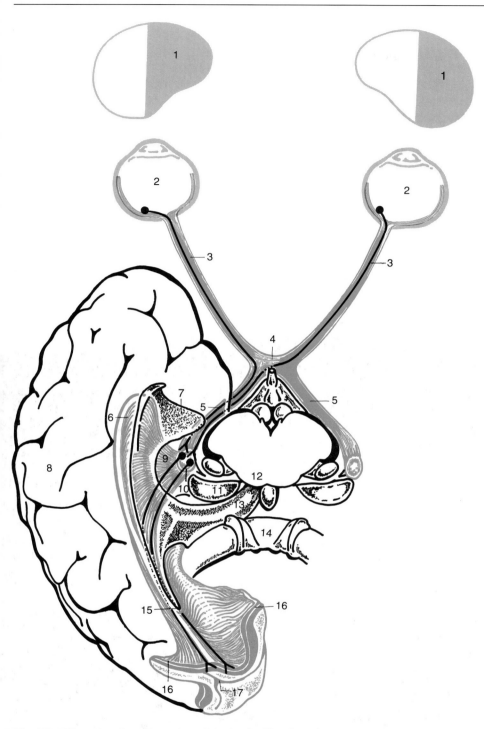

1 Corresponding halves of visual field
2 Ocular bulb
3 Optic nerve
4 Optic chiasm
5 Optic tract
6 Temporal genu of optic radiation
7 Temporal horn of lateral ventricle
8 Temporal lobe of cerebrum
9 Optic radiation
10 Lateral geniculate body
11 Pulvinar of thalamus
12 Superior colliculus
13 Central part of lateral ventricle
14 Splenium of corpus callosum
15 Occipital horn of lateral ventricle
16 Visual cortex
17 Calcarine sulcus

Fig. 53 The visual system (caudal view). The basal parts of the diencephalon and mesencephalon are located between the optic tracts. The temporal and occipital lobes are the only portions of the right telencephalon shown. Two homonymous halves of the visual field are shown in gray. The path of the neurons from one half of the retina to the respective visual cortex is shown. According to (206).

1 Retina
2 Optic nerve
3 Optic chiasm

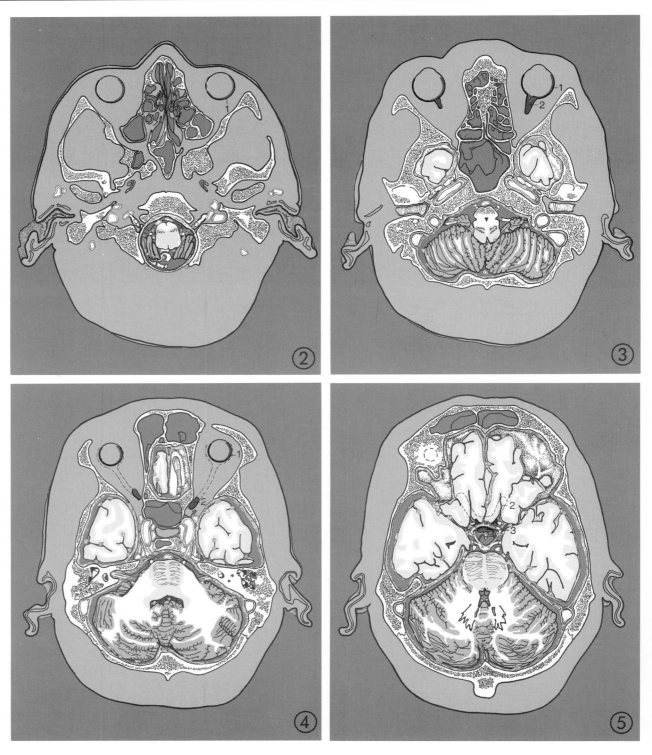

Fig. 54 Serial illustrations of the visual system. The encircled number indicates the number of the respective slice (see Figs. 1a, 2, 3, 4).

3 Optic chiasm
4 Optic tract
5 Lateral geniculate body
6 Optic radiation
7 Visual cortex

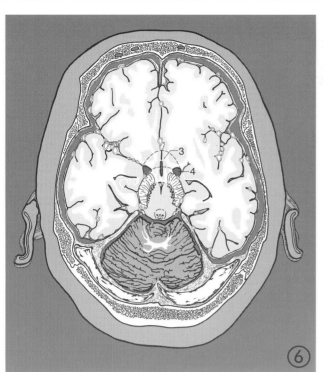

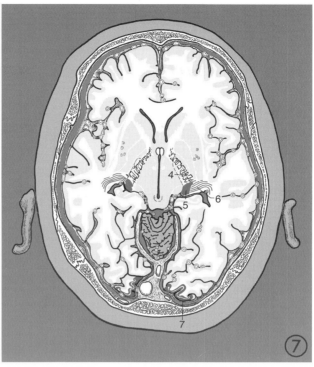

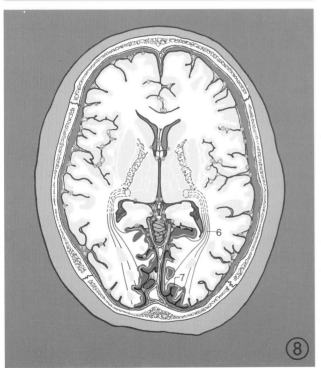

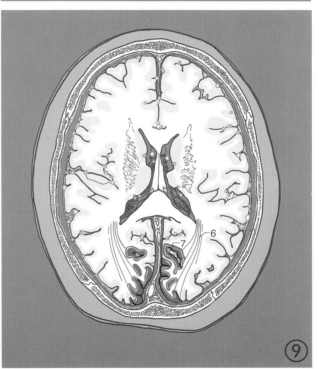

Point-to-point projections exist between the photo-receptors of the retina and the visual cortex:

1. As a result of the partial crossing of the optic nerve fibers in the optic chiasm, the optic signals arising from the right halves of both retinae (the left halves of the visual fields) reach the right visual cortex.
2. The lower homonymous quadrants of the retina (the upper homonymous quadrants of the visual field) project into the portion of the visual cortex located below the calcarine sulcus (the lower lip of the visual cortex). The upper retinal quadrants project to the cortex above the calcarine sulcus.
3. The macula lutea, the region of most acute sight, maintains the largest field of projection in the visual cortex. This field is located at the occipital pole of the brain. The visual cortex of the peripheral binocular visual field lies ventral to the occipital pole, and that of the peripheral monocular visual field is situated close to the parieto-occipital sulcus.

In addition to this major pathway of the optic nerve, there is also a small extrageniculate supplementary pathway which most likely could partially compensate for deficits of the major pathway. This extrageniculate projection bypasses the lateral geniculate body and reaches the superior colliculi and the pulvinar of the thalamus. From this thalamic nucleus, optic signals are transmitted to the primary and secondary visual cortices (222, 233, 280).

As satisfactory examination of the retina can be accomplished with an ophthalmoscope; further examinations are seldom necessary. Additional studies are only called for if a lesion of the posterior section of the eyeball or retrobulbar space is suspected. Clinical indications of a retrobulbar disorder may include visual disturbances in one eye, pain upon movement of the eye, protrusio bulbi (forward projection of the eyeball), and chemosis (edema of the ocular conjunctiva). Pathological changes and functional disorders of the optic nerve as well as processes in the retrobulbar space are indications for the use of computed tomography. The reclining position of the head (preferred for this CT examination) sets the sectioning plane at 10° to the canthomeatal plane. This corresponds approximately to the infraorbitomeatal plane (199, 235). The optic nerve, the straight muscles, and the maximal circumference of the eyeball are clearly imaged and constantly reproducible in this plane (313).

CT shows alterations of the optic nerve and pathological densities in the retrobulbar space. The diameter of the optic nerve can be determined exactly by choosing a coronal plane as the sectioning plane (235, 313). In cases involving minimal functional disorders of the optic nerve, especially status post optic nerve neuritis, the determination of the VEP (Visually Evoked Potentials) is a sensitive diagnostic procedure.

Disorders in the region of the optic chiasm may result in bitemporal and, less frequently, in binasal hemianopsia. Enlargement of the sella turcica or, more rarely, destruction of the sella turcica may appear in lateral X-rays of the skull. CT scans establish pathological density patterns in the region of the optic chiasm and may occasionally identify bony destructions in the region of the sella turcica (pituitary fossa). Lesions in the optic tract and/or lateral geniculate body may result in a contralateral homonymous hemianopsia.

Homonymous quadrantanopsia and homonymous hemianopsia are clinical symptoms indicating a pathological process in the region of the optic radiation or primary visual cortex. Furthermore, symptoms of irritation such as photopsia and amaurosis fugax may be seen. Bilateral vascular or traumatic injuries affecting the visual cortex may result in cortical blindness.

4.7 Olfactory System (Figs. 55 and 63)

In the upper and posterior part of the nasal cavity just below the cribriform plate of the ethmoid bone lies the olfactory epithelium. This area of 2 cm² contains the olfactory receptors. Approximately twenty olfactory fila arise in each side from the olfactory neurosensory cells of the nose and extend through the cribriform plate. The first neurons terminate in the olfactory bulb forming several synaptic brushlike terminals or olfactory glomeruli. These synaptic glomeruli establish contact with the mitral cells. On the average, the human olfactory bulb is 10 mm long, 4.5 mm wide, and flattened in the vertical plane (271). It is considerably smaller than that of apes (289).

The axons of the mitral cells form the olfactory tract. This extends into small cortical areas at the base of the telencephalon (paleocortex) and is divided into medial and lateral olfactory striae. The medial olfactory stria extends toward a center below the genu of the corpus callosum corresponding to the olfactory trigone of macrosmatic animals. The lateral olfactory stria extends laterally, bending sharply around the edge of the insula, and projecting into the periamygdaloid cortex and prepiriform cortex of the gyrus semilunaris (290) (Fig. 10b.15). These small cortical areas lie hidden in the angular space between the temporal lobe and the neighboring edge of the insula. The periamygdaloid cortex is part of the amygdaloid body. The olfactory tract extends uncrossed to the ipsilateral cerebral cortex. The olfactory centers on both sides are connected by the anterior commissure.

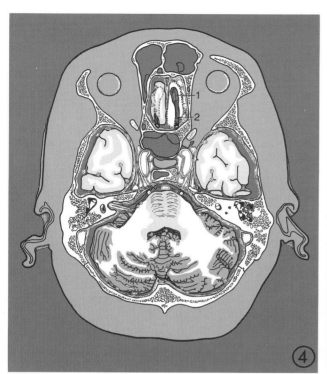

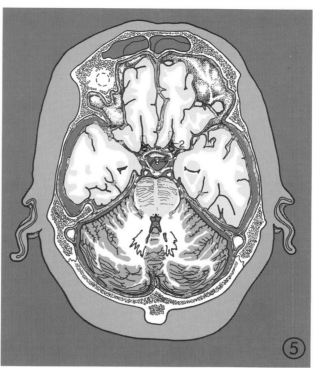

1 Olfactory bulb
2 Olfactory tract
3 Olfactory trigone (within the slice)
4 Prepiriform and periamygdaloid cortical areas (partial within the slice)

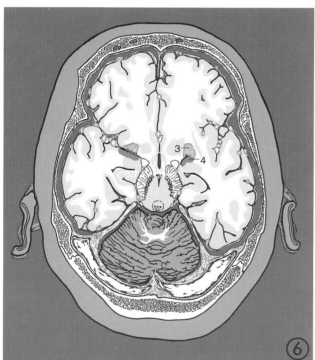

Fig. 55 Serial illustrations of the olfactory system. The encircled number indicates the number of the respective slice (see Figs. 1a, 2, 3, 4).

A loss of the sense of smell results in a subjective impairment of the sense of taste. This is probably accounted for by the common cortical processing of olfactory and gustatory signals. Disturbances of olfaction arise as a result of injury to the olfactory epithelium or damage to the olfactory nerves and/or bulbs. Unilateral impairment is noticed seldom spontaneously by the patient. Olfactory hallucinations can arise due to lesions in the region of the olfactory tract and as a symptom of temporal lobe epilepsy (uncinate seizure).

4.8 Motor Systems

Cortical and subcortical neurons are joined by synapses with the motor neurons of the midbrain, pons, medulla oblongata, and spinal cord (164, 165, 166). Anatomical and physiological research over the past few decades has shown that the cortical and subcortical nerve cells are closely linked by numerous feedback loops. This research has led to a revision of the classical concept of two totally separate motor systems, namely the pyramidal (voluntary) system and the extrapyramidal (involuntary) system (155). Daily activities, such as swinging the arms while walking or running, illustrate the connection between voluntary and automatic movements. Voluntary movement, therefore, is actually a sort of voluntary/involuntary mixture. In accordance with this concept, the pyramidal pathway provides a significant route for output signals arising from individual systems of the basal ganglia, such as the striatothalamic main circuits.

Neuropathological investigations and clinical examinations usually associate neurological symptoms with the pyramidal system or with specific systems of the basal ganglia. The Babinski reflex, for instance, may be seen as a result of a disorder in the pyramidal pathway or akinesia due to a lesion in the substantia nigra. For this reason, we will maintain the notion of a pyramidal system. The individual motor systems of the basal ganglia, however, will be treated separately.

Detections of disorders in the motor systems are of primary importance in clinical diagnosis. In many cases involving unconscious or only partially cooperative patients, an adequate test of motor signs is still possible. Often motor disorders are so obvious that a simple test is sufficient for an approximate topical localization of the insult. Therefore, the preparation of more specific diagnostic or therapeutic measures is possible, before a subtle evaluation of the patient's conditions might be accomplished.

Damage to the so-called "upper motor neurons" is characterized by paralysis, loss of polysynaptic reflexes (e.g., superficial abdominal reflexes), and the appearance of pathological reflexes of the Babinski group. An increase in the tonus (spasticity)

of the paralyzed extremities develops at variable rates. Finally, a typical clinical picture can be described, whereby a distally accentuated paralysis and a typical posture appear. Characteristic symptoms of a hemiplegic patient are the circumduction of the paralyzed leg and the adduction and flexion of the paralyzed arm (Wernicke-Mann's syndrome).

4.8.1 Pyramidal System (Figs. 56 and 57)

The pyramidal system originates in pyramidal cells of the cerebral cortex. These cells are located anterior and posterior to the central sulcus in and around the precentral and postcentral gyri. Cytoarchitectonically, this primarily includes areas 2 and 6, also areas 3, 1, 4, and 5, in which regions like the primary motor cortex, the supplementary motor, and the somatic sensory areas are located (57, 106, 173).

The primary motor cortex exhibits a fine somatotopic organization. Located on the medial surface of the hemisphere are the upper motor neurons that supply the spinal motor neurons of the leg muscles. Cortical regions responsible for innervation of the trunk, arm, facial, masticatory, lingual, and laryngeal muscles extend from the superior margin toward the lateral sulcus. The lower motor neurons receive their input contralaterally. Additional ipsilateral innervation is received by the lower motor neurons of the muscles of the eyes, mandible, larynx, and upper face (occipitofrontalis and orbicularis oculi muscles). The supplementary motor area lies between area 4 and the paralimbic mesocortex on the medial surface of the hemisphere (28). A crude somatotopic organization is recognizable.

The corticonuclear fibers extend from the motor cortex to the motor neurons of the cranial nerves. The corticospinal fibers connect the motor cortex with the motor neurons of the spinal cord. Both pathways can have interposed interneurons that are located at the same level as the motor neurons.

The corticonuclear fibers descend through the genu of the internal capsule, pass through the cerebral peduncles, and reach the motor nuclei of the V, VII, IX, X, XII, and XI (partially) cranial nerves in the tegmentum of the pons and medulla oblongata. According to new research, the corticonuclear and corticospinal fibers are located in the dorsal part of the posterior limb of the internal capsule (66, 98, 99, 100, 251), although this view is not accepted unanimously (253). Underway, the pathways cross to the opposite side and terminate directly or indirectly via interneurons on the lower motor neurons. The majority of the cranial nerve motor nuclei (V, IX, and X) receive additional input from the ipsilateral motor cortex and, therefore, are bilaterally innervated. The motor nuclei of the eleventh and twelfth cranial nerves receive their input from the contra-

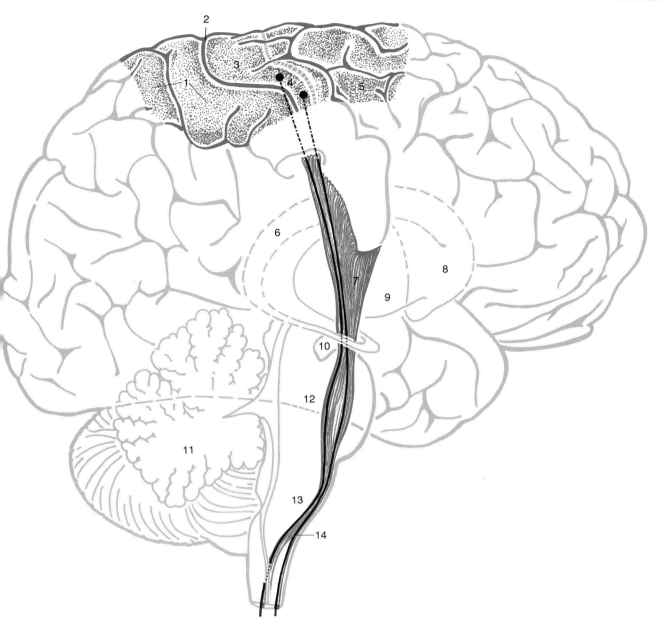

Fig. 56 The pyramidal (corticospinal) tract (lateral view). The origin of the pyramidal (corticospinal) tract in the telencephalic cortex and the long corticofugal system are shown transparently. The brain stem and cerebellum are dissected in the median plane. The right half of both structures has been removed with exception of the pyramidal (corticospinal) tract and the substantia nigra. According to (206).

1 Lateral corticospinal tract
2 Anterior corticospinal tract
3 Corticospinal tract

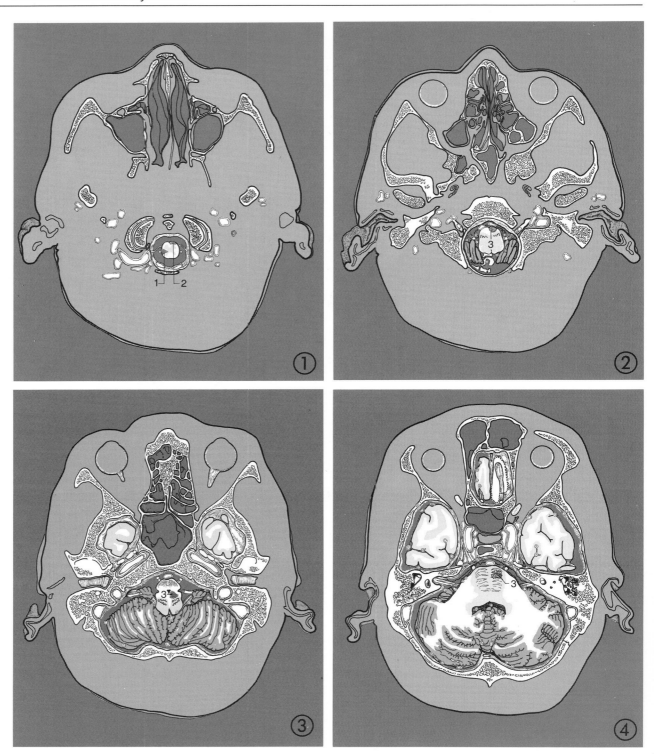

Fig. 57 Serial illustrations of the pyramidal (corticospinal) tract and its areas of origin. The encircled number indicates the number of the respective slice (see Figs. 1a, 2, 3, 4).

3 Corticospinal tract

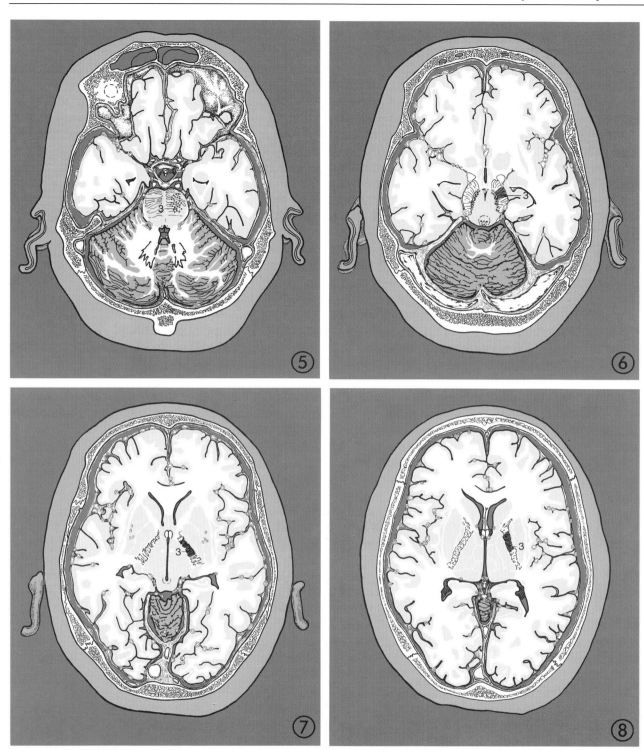

3 Corticospinal tract
4 Precentral gyrus
5 Premotor cortex
6 Sensorimotor cortex
7 Paracentral lobule

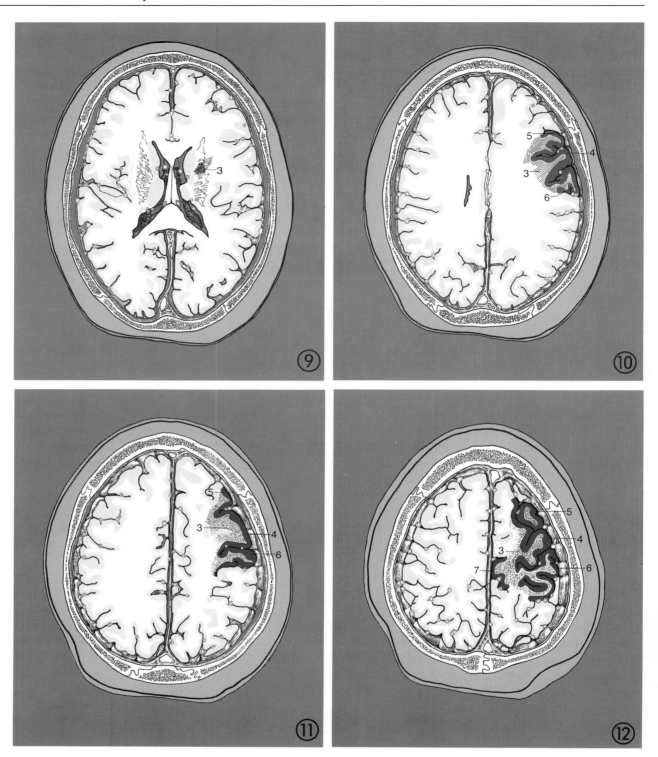

Fig. 57   Serial illustrations of the pyramidal (corticospinal) tract and its areas of origin. The encircled number indicates the number of the respective slice (see Figs. 1a, 2, 3, 4).

3 Corticospinal tract
4 Precentral gyrus
5 Premotor cortex
6 Sensorimotor cortex
7 Paracentral lobule

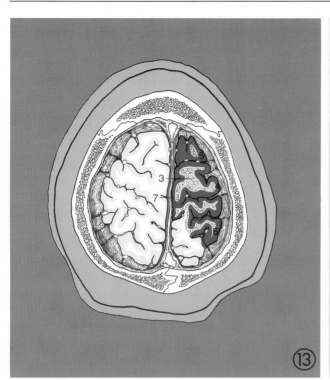

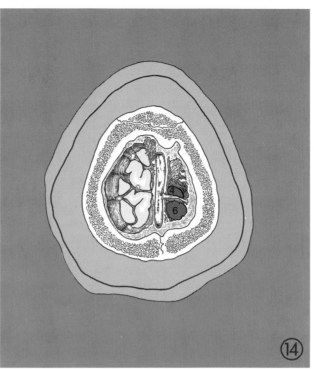

lateral cerebral cortex alone. The motor nucleus of the facial nerve has two differently innervated regions. The motor neurons of the occipitofrontalis and the orbicularis oculi muscles receive inputs via both ipsilateral and contralateral connections. The remaining muscles of facial expression are innervated contralaterally only.

Knowledge of these two sources of innervation for the motor nucleus of the facial nerve is necessary when distinguishing facial paralysis of the upper or lower motor neuron. A lesion of the corticonuclear fibers in the internal capsule on one side caused by a hemorrhage, for example, results in a contralateral paralysis of all muscles of facial expression except for the occipitofrontalis and the orbicularis oculi muscles. In other words, although the patient with a unilateral lesion is able to wrinkle the forehead on the side contralateral to the hemorrhage, the cheek and oral muscles of the face are paretic (weak) (supranuclear paresis of the upper motor neuron). Injury to the facial nucleus or nerve on one side, results in a paralysis of all of the facial (mimetic) muscles on that side (nuclear/infranuclear paralysis of the lower motor neuron).

The corticospinal fibers (pyramidal pathway) transmit motor impulses to the contralateral spinal motor neurons (317). Originating in the somatotopically organized regions of the cerebral cortex, the axons of large and small pyramidal cells extend through the internal capsule, the cerebral peduncles, the basal portion of the pons, and the medulla oblongata. Here the pyramidal pathways form bilateral, cord-like elevations – the pyramids – hence the name. Immediately above the spinal cord, about 75% of the fibers cross at the pyramidal decussation and form the lateral corticospinal tract. This tract descends the entire length of the lateral funiculus. The smaller uncrossed portion of the pyramidal pathway, located in the anterior funiculus, descends as the anterior corticospinal tract to the middle of the thoracic spinal cord. It crosses at the top of the corresponding spinal segment. The interneurons, which act as relays between the pyramidal pathway and the spinal motor neurons, are usually connected with numerous motor neurons or form parts of inhibitory feedback loops.

The somatotopic division of the motor cortex with its relatively wide divergence of the corticonuclear and corticospinal tracts explains the frequent appearance of incomplete paralyses or of monopareses in patients having lesions in and around the motor cortex. Irritative processes in the motor cortex may lead to focal epileptic seizures.

The tight bundling of all motor fibers of one hemisphere in the internal capsule accounts for extensive contralateral hemiplegia observed as a result of a lesion in the internal capsule. The topographical proximity of the motor pathways to the terminal part of the sensory pathway in the posterior portion of the internal capsule accounts for simultaneous hemisensory disorders in cases of hemiplegia. Lesions of the posterior portion of the internal capsule may damage the optic pathway and result in a homonymous hemianopsia of the opposite side.

A hemiplegia with supranuclear facial paralysis and eye muscle disorders indicates a lesion in the midbrain and/or the dorsal part of the pons (pars dorsalis tegmenti pontis). Injuries affecting pons and medulla oblongata are a cause of both ipsilateral cranial nerve disorders accompanied by swallowing and speech impairment (cranial nerves IX, X, and XII) and contralateral hemiplegias (crossed syndromes).

4.8.2 Motor Systems of the Basal Ganglia (Fig. 58)

The motor systems of the basal ganglia are composed of subcortical groups of nuclei. These nuclei have extensive connections with the motor cortex of the telencephalon and form several loops or circuits among themselves (155). In accordance with these neuronal loops, it appears that the neurons of the basal ganglia form several control circuits. The neurons receive their input from the reticular formation, cerebellar, and cortical regions. The output leaves primarily via the pyramidal pathway but descending multisynaptic pathways, such as the reticulospinal and vestibulospinal pathways, also carry efferent signals.

The main structures comprising the motor systems of the basal ganglia, are the striatum (putamen and caudate nucleus), globus pallidus, subthalamic nucleus, and substantia nigra. Stereotactic operations have shown that small nuclei of the lateral thalamic nucleus, namely the ventral anterior and ventral lateral nuclei, can significantly influence rigidity and tremor (105). For this reason, these smaller nuclei may also be considered part of the basal ganglia.

Important afferent signals reaching the basal ganglia arrive in the striatum from the reticular formation via small thalamic nuclei, such as the intralaminar nuclei. Pathways project from the dentate nucleus in the cerebellum via the ventral lateral nucleus of the thalamus, to the pallidum and the motor cortex. The mesostriatal serotoninergic system, whose cell bodies lie in the dorsal raphe nucleus of the midbrain, terminates in the striatum.

The main transmission circuit of the basal ganglia originates in the neocortex, extends to the striatum, and projects via the globus pallidus into the ventral anterior and ventral lateral nuclei of the thalamus. These nuclei project to the motor and premotor cortex (areas 4 and 6). Apparently, this loop "collects" information from the entire neocortex and processes it for the motor and premotor cortex.

In addition, three supplementary circuits connect the

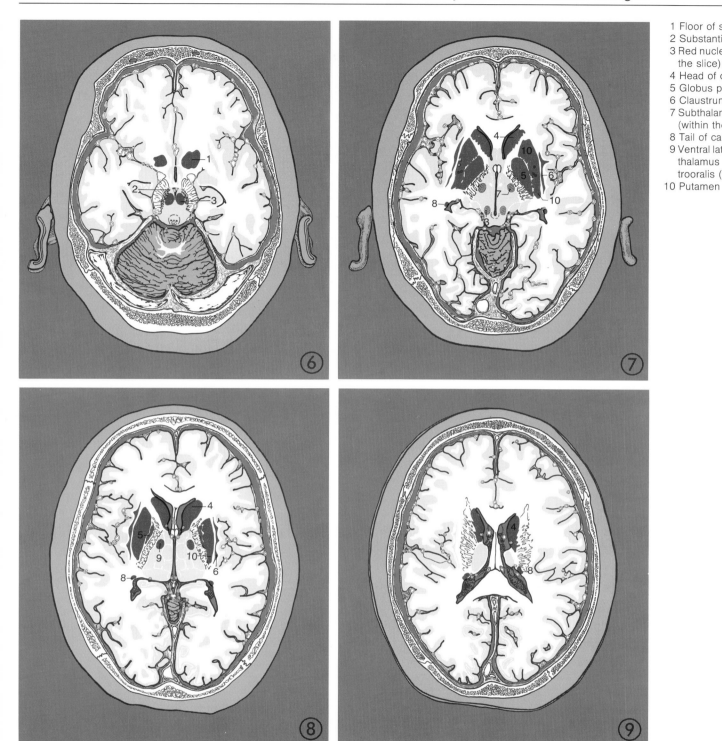

1 Floor of striatum
2 Substantia nigra
3 Red nucleus (partial within the slice)
4 Head of caudate nucleus
5 Globus pallidus
6 Claustrum
7 Subthalamic nucleus (within the slice)
8 Tail of caudate nucleus
9 Ventral lateral nucleus of thalamus (nucleus ventrooralis (107))
10 Putamen

Fig. 58 Serial illustrations of the basal ganglia. The encircled number indicates the number of the respective slice (see Figs. 1a, 2, 3, 4).

previously mentioned nuclei of the basal ganglia. In these circuits, the striatum assumes a central role.

The first supplementary loop extends from the striatum to the globus pallidus, then to the centromedian nucleus of the thalamus, and back to the striatum. The second loop projects from the globus pallidus to the subthalamic nucleus and back. The third supplementary loop (striatum → substantia nigra → striatum) uses two different transmitter substances: GABA and dopamine. The striatonigral fibers use GABA, the nigrostriatal fibers are dopaminergic.

Disorders of the basal ganglia cause characteristic changes in motor functions including speech. Such changes may be obvious as spontaneous hyperkinesia, tonus changes (especially rigidity), hypokinesia, tremor, and characteristic postural disorders. In hereditary Huntington's chorea, the severity of the clinical symptoms, hyperkinesia and dementia, often correlates with the widened ventricles as seen in CT scans, which demonstrate typical atrophy of the caudate nucleus and putamen and also a diffuse, subcortically accentuated brain atrophy.

In cases of Parkinson's syndrome, CT scans provide few consistent pathological findings. In addition to infrequent abnormal findings, dilatations of the ventricles and subarachnoid spaces are quite common. Parkinson's syndrome is generally recognized as a disorder of the dopaminergic system (Chap. 4.12.1). Athetosis arises as a result of non-uniform anatomical lesions. CT findings, therefore, also vary considerably. Hemiballism (uncontrollable flailing movements of one or both limbs on the contralateral side) is often associated with vascular disorders in the subthalamic nucleus or its connections.

The corticonuclear and corticospinal fibers are important efferent pathways of the basal ganglia. These fibers originate in the motor and premotor cortex and receive an input from the main striatal loop. There is uncertainty, however, about the number of motor signals that are transmitted downward parallel to the pyramidal pathways. Parallel projections, originating in the basal ganglia, extend via the substantia nigra to the tectum and the reticular formation. The tectospinal and reticulospinal tracts descend from here into the spinal cord. Descending fibers of the lateral vestibular nucleus, such as the lateral vestibulospinal tract, belong to the output system of the basal ganglia as well. Fiber bundles connect the basal ganglia with the limbic system. The pallidohabenular fibers connect the medial segment of the pallidum with a portion of the limbic system (lateral habenular nucleus).

4.8.3 Oculomotor System

The oculomotor system controls movements of the extraocular muscles by way of the third, fourth, and sixth cranial nerves. Oculomotor disorders are important in clinical diagnosis. Conjugate gaze paralyses, impaired pupillary motor activities, paralyses of convergence, nystagmus, and paralyses of the third, fourth, and sixth cranial nerves are obvious symptoms. A neurological examination frequently suffices to locate the lesion (152).

Two cortical areas of the telencephalon, that are not part of the pyramidal motor cortex, are responsible for the movements of the eyes. These two cortical areas are composed of a small frontal region and a large occipital region. The frontal cortical area is located in the posterior portion of the middle frontal gyrus and corresponds to Brodmann's area 8. It controls voluntary eye movements independent of visual stimuli. The frontal cortical area constantly triggers the eye muscles to scan the visual field. The occipital cortical area corresponds to areas 17, 18, and 19. Area 17 simultaneously acts as the cortical projection field for the optic radiation. The occipital cortical areas control eye movements resulting from visual stimuli.

The ocular corticofugal pathways, originating in the frontal and occipital cortical areas are not directly connected with the motor neurons but project first to the superior colliculus and the pretectal area (163). In their subsequent course, preoculomotor centers including the interstitial nucleus (Cajal), parts of the paramedian pontine reticular formation (parabducens nucleus), and the prepositus hypoglossal nucleus are further relay centers. These intermediary neuron systems coordinate the conjugate movements of both eyes.

The motor nuclei of the third and fourth cranial nerves are located in the tegmentum of the midbrain (Figs. 36.10 and 36.11), the abducens nucleus is situated in the pontine tegmentum (Fig. 36.14).

In cases of conjugate gaze palsy, conjugate horizontal or vertical movements of the eyes are either impaired or are completely nonfunctional. Paralysis of conjugate eye movements is always supranuclear. Diplopia (double vision) is not usually associated with conjugate gaze paralysis. Disconjugate paralysis impairs the convergence and divergence movements of the eyes.

Horizontal conjugate gaze paralysis is generally temporary in cases of cerebral lesions with unilateral interruption of the corticopontine control pathways. A lesion in the frontal eye field causes an inability to move the eyes voluntarily to the opposite side. Instead, the conjugate gaze may drift to the side of the lesion. This lesion is especially obvious in unconscious patients. Irritation (e.g., epilepsy) leads to a seizure-like onset of contraversive gaze. Pontine lesions may cause conjugate gaze paralysis with deviation to the side opposite of the lesion.

Gaze paralysis in the vertical plane arises with lesions located near the superior colliculi. Upward gaze paralysis is far more frequent than downward. Vertical gaze paralysis in combination with convergence paralysis is known as Parinaud's syndrome and is typically seen in patients with pineal region tumors. Internuclear ophthalmoplegia appears as a result of a lesion in the medial longitudinal fasciculus with interruption of the connections between the abducens nuclei or the oculomotor nuclei. This results in a motility impairment to one side of one or both eyes. When looking straight ahead, the patient experiences no double vision. Such disorders may arise with multiple sclerosis and vascular lesions (270).

Double vision is the guideline symptom for disorders of the lower motor neurons of the nerves controlling the eye muscles. In the absence of further neurological symptoms, it is difficult to differentiate clinically between myogenic and neurogenic paresis. Nuclear and infranuclear injuries have to be considered in cases of neurogenic lesions. The patient's history and further localizing symptoms are decisive in making a diagnosis.

Likewise, infranuclear paresis of the ocular muscles and impairment of the ophthalmic division of the trigeminal nerve are part of the superior orbital fissure syndrome. A syndrome of the orbit apex can be classified as an advanced superior orbital fissure syndrome. In addition to the symptoms mentioned, impairments of the optic nerve, ophthalmic artery, and orbital veins will be seen.

Pupillary anomalies play an important role in clinical diagnosis. Pupils, which are abnormally dilated on both sides, are found in association with midbrain lesions. Abnormally small pupils indicate foci in the pons. Unequal abnormalities in pupillary size appear with unilateral mydriasis (oculomotor paresis – frequently with ptosis and impaired motility of the eyes) or unilateral miosis (Horner's syndrome is a combination of miosis with ptosis and enophthalmos of the same side). Abnormal pupillary reactions may be caused by optic nerve lesions (iridoplegia), an oculomotor nerve injury or, more frequently, by a lesion of the eyeball.

4.9 Cerebellar Systems (Figs. 59, 60, 61)

The cerebellum receives afferent pathways from virtually all receptors in the human body (33, 63). These include, among others, proprioceptive, exteroceptive, vestibular, auditory, and visual receptors. The cerebral cortex projects via the pontine nuclei and through pontocerebellar tracts into the cerebellum. The corticopontocerebellar pathways extend through the massive middle cerebellar peduncle. Most of the efferent pathways originate in the cerebellar nuclei and mainly leave the cerebellum via the superior cerebellar peduncles. The ratio of afferent fibers in the cerebellum to efferent fibers is 40:1 (112). This input: output ratio explains the substantial coordinative role assumed by the cerebellum for all motor functions from standing and walking to speaking and writing.

The cerebellar pathways are connected with the archeo-, paleo-, and neocerebellum. The nodule of vermis, flocculus, and fastigial nucleus are considered parts of the archeocerebellum. The afferent archeocerebellar pathway is the vestibulocerebellar tract. It consists of direct fibers from the vestibular portion of the eighth cranial nerve and axons from the vestibular nuclei. The vestibulocerebellar tract ends in the flocculonodular lobe and in the fastigial nucleus. This pathway extends through the inferior cerebellar peduncle. The efferent archeocortical pathway, the cerebellovestibular tract, extends through the inferior cerebellar peduncle to each of the vestibular nuclei with exception of the lateral vestibular nucleus (308). For this reason, the archeocerebellum is also called vestibulocerebellum (33). Lesions in the archeocerebellum lead to disorders of bilateral movement and impaired regulation of equilibrium with entire trunk, stationary, and gait ataxia without additional cerebellar symptoms (10, 41, 230). The patient's gait is similar to the swaying, staggering movements of drunks.

The anterior lobe, the pyramis of vermis, and the uvula of vermis are parts of the paleocerebellum. The anterior and posterior spinocerebellar tracts and a pathway from a nucleus of the posterior funiculus, the cuneate nucleus (Burdach), terminate in this part of the cerebellar cortex. The cuneocerebellar tract passes through the inferior cerebellar peduncle, mainly into the anterior lobe, but also contributes to the posterior lobe. The posterior spinocerebellar tract extends through the inferior cerebellar peduncle and the anterior spinocerebellar tract through the superior cerebellar peduncle to the paleocerebellum. During evolution, the neocerebellar pathways migrated as the middle cerebellar peduncle between the spinocerebellar pathways. Due to its numerous afferent connections originating in the spinal cord, the paleocerebellum is also referred to as spinocerebellum (33). This does not take into

1 Tonsil of cerebellum,
  neocerebellum
2 Flocculus,
  archeocerebellum
3 Posterior lobe,
  neocerebellum
4 Uvula of vermis,
  paleocerebellum
5 Pyramis of vermis,
  paleocerebellum
6 Anterior lobe,
  paleocerebellum
7 Nodule of vermis,
  archeocerebellum

Neocerebellum
Paleocerebellum
Archeocerebellum

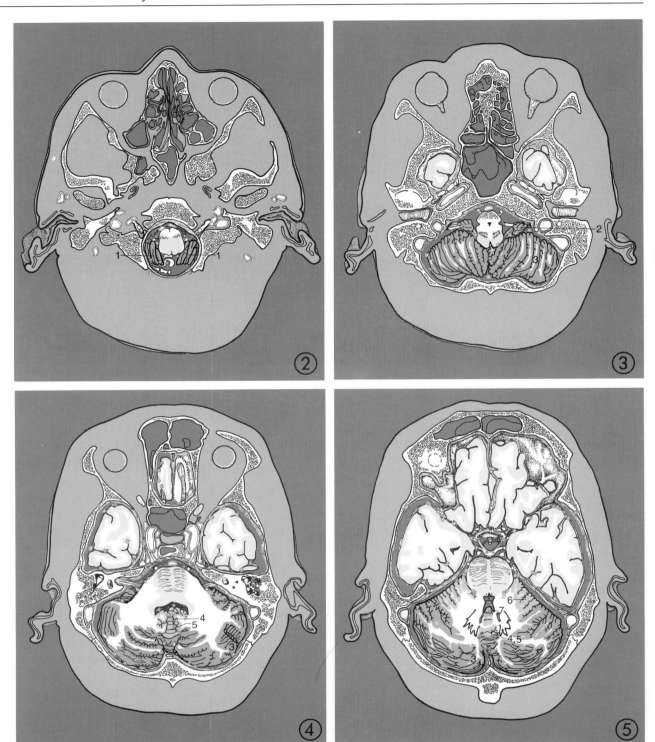

Fig. 59 Serial illustrations of the cerebellar cortical areas. The encircled number indicates the number of the respective slice (see Figs. 1a, 2, 3, 4).

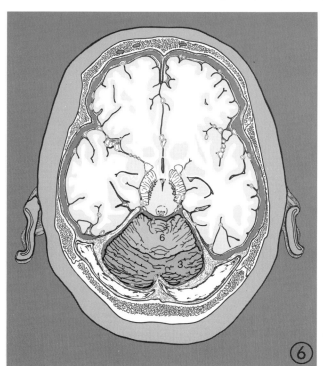

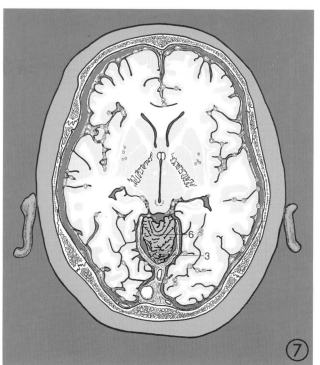

3 Posterior lobe,
  neocerebellum
6 Anterior lobe,
  paleocerebellum

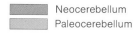 Neocerebellum
               Paleocerebellum

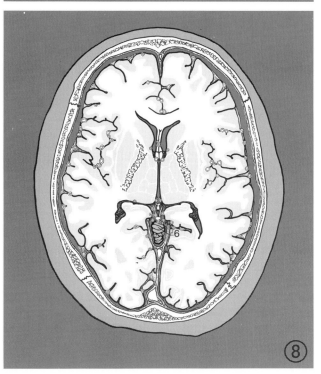

1 Thalamus
2 Corticopontine tract
3 Red nucleus
4 Tectum of mesencephalon
5 Decussation of superior
  cerebellar peduncles
6 Superior cerebellar
  peduncle
7 Vermis of anterior lobe of
  cerebellum
8 Anterior spinocerebellar
  tract
9 Primary fissure
10 Pons
11 Trigeminal nerve
12 Pontocerebellar tract
13 Inferior cerebellar
   peduncle
14 Middle cerebellar
   peduncle
15 Inferior olivary nucleus
16 Olivocerebellar tract
17 Hemisphere of posterior
   lobe
18 External arcuate fibers
19 Posterior spinocerebellar
   tract

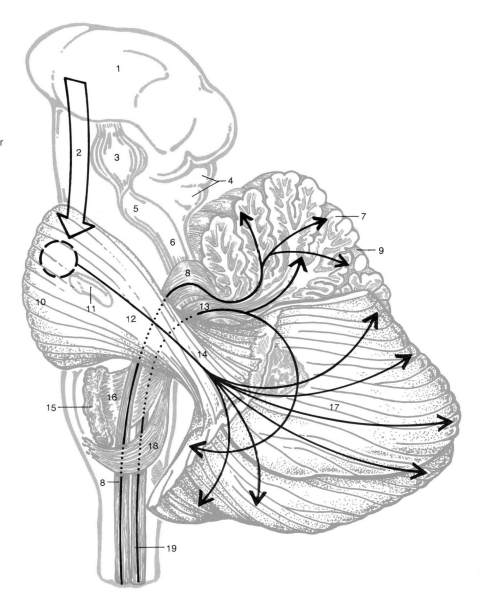

Fig. 60 The afferent systems of the cerebellum (lateral view). The left half of the anterior lobe of the cerebellum and the archeocerebellum have been removed. According to (206).

1 Motor and premotor cortex
  (area 4 and 6)
2 Pyramidal tract
3 Ventral lateral nucleus of
  thalamus
4 Ventral anterior nucleus of
  thalamus
5 Red nucleus
6 Superior cerebellar
  peduncle
7 Purkinje cells
8 Dentate nucleus
9 Fastigial nucleus
10 Vestibular nuclei

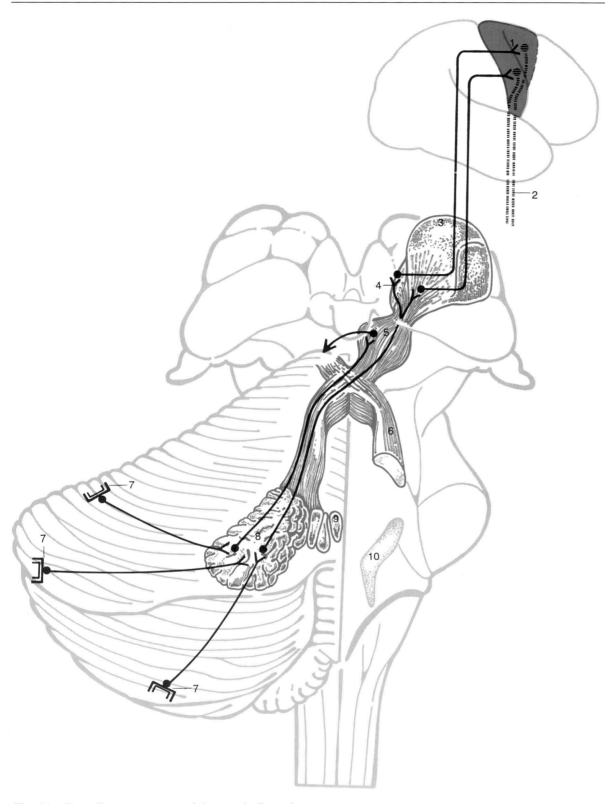

Fig. 61 The efferent systems of the cerebellum showing the location of the pathways and the nuclei (dorsal view). The cerebellum has been dissected in the median plane, and the entire right half has been removed with the exception of the superior cerebellar peduncle. According to (206).

account that the olivocerebellar tract projects into the entire cerebellar cortex (41).

The neocerebellum develops between the phylogenetically older parts of the cerebellum. Neocortical pathways originate mainly from the frontal and temporal cerebral cortices and, to a lesser extent, from the parietal and occipital cortices and extend via the cerebral peduncles to the pontine nuclei. The relay to the pontocerebellar tract takes place here. The majority of the fibers cross to the opposite side of the neocerebellum or to the cerebellar nuclei. A small portion of the pontocerebellar fibers projects to the paleocerebellum (41). The existence of the tectocerebellar tract has recently been questioned (33). Signals emitted from the tectum appear to reach the cerebellum via the pontine nuclei.

The efferent pathways of the neocerebellum extend primarily to the dentate nucleus. The axons of the next group of neurons pass through the superior cerebellar peduncle, cross in the lower midbrain, and reach the red nucleus, reticular formation, and ventral anterior and ventral lateral nuclei of the thalamus. The thalamic nuclei project to the motor cortex. Due to the decussation of the efferent cerebellar pathways in the midbrain and, as a consequence of the redecussation of the pyramidal pathways, each cerebellar hemisphere is connected with the ipsilateral spinal cord. Unilateral cerebellar lesions, therefore, lead to ipsilateral dysfunctions. Neocerebellar lesions are characterized by impaired motor coordination. In cases of cerebellar ataxia, the muscles involved fail to work in harmony even when the patient uses visual control. In finger-to-nose testing, intention tremor will appear even with the eyes open. Rapid repetition of movements is not possible (adiadochokinesis). Goal oriented movement is incorrectly estimated (dysmetria). Speech is often choppy (the typical disorder being scanning dysarthria). Muscle tonus may be decreased (hypotonia of the musculature). A nystagmus is sometimes observed when the patient glances toward the side of the injured cerebellar hemisphere.

4.10 Language Areas (Fig. 62)

The language areas were first localized by two clinicians, namely Broca in 1861 and Wernicke in 1874. Up to now, it has been impossible to identify specific nerve cells or synapses which are unique to the language areas of the dominant hemisphere. Diagnosis of aphasia, therefore, must be made in living patients. As a result, such research is dominated by clinicians and linguists. Aphasia is different from disorders of speech resulting from weakness or incoordination of the muscles that control the vocal apparatus. These are referred to as dysarthria (diffi-

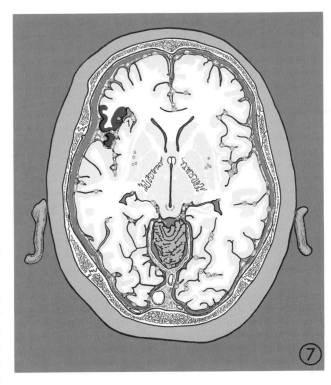

culty in articulation) and dysphonia (difficulty in vocalization).

Language areas are lateralized in one hemisphere and, in at least 95% of all individuals, this is the left hemisphere (86). Greater than 99% of all right-handed individuals have a languagedominant left hemisphere. In left-handed persons a dominance of the left hemisphere is present in about 60%. In some left-handed individuals a bilateral representation of language areas is thought to exist (14).

Language disorders are usually the result of an occluded blood vessel (86, 147, 176, 231). This means that the pathological lesion may be larger than the actual language area. Without morphological criteria, the exact location of the affected language area cannot be pinpointed. For this reason, it is understandable that different topical descriptions of the language areas have been published. In Figure 62, the boundaries of three language areas are drawn according to the minimal size of the areas as given in the references (86, 147, 176, 231).

Broca's (motor) area is damaged by an occlusion of the artery to the precentral sulcus (231) (Prerolandic artery (128)). Broca's area occupies the operculum of the inferior frontal gyrus. Based on cytoarchitectonic criteria, this area corresponds to Brodmann's area 44 (62). Analysis of CT scans shows additional involvement of the neighboring insular region (24).

Wernicke's (sensory) area lies in the superior temporal gyrus between the primary auditory cortex and the angular gyrus. This area is supplied by the pos-

1 Broca's area
2 Wernicke's area
3 Angular gyrus

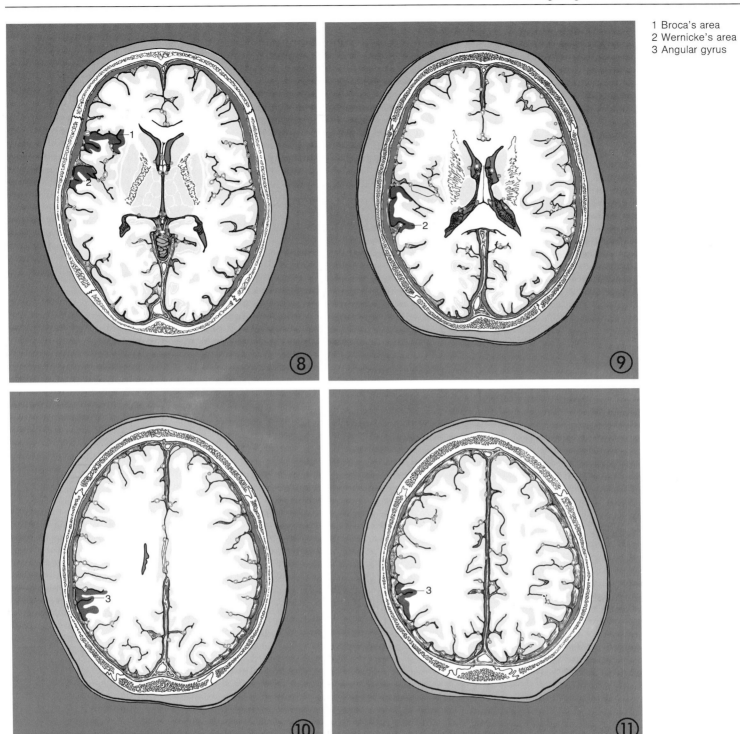

Fig. 62   Serial illustrations of the language areas. The encircled number indicates the number of the respective slice (see Figs. 1a, 2, 3, 4).

terior temporal artery which arises from the medial cerebral artery (231). The visual auditory conversion language area is located in the angular gyrus (86). The language areas lie alongside the corresponding primary cortices of the neocortex. Broca's area lies in the frontal lobe, rostral to the primary motor cortex. Wernicke's area is located between the primary auditory, visual, and sensory cortices, in other words, between the transverse temporal gyri (Heschl), visual cortex, and postcentral gyrus. Expressive (motor or nonfluent) aphasia usually arises from a lesion of Broca's area with limited language comprehension and agrammatism. Receptive (sensory or fluent) aphasia is characterized by a loss of language comprehension and a lesion of Wernicke's area.

Besides cortical lesions, subcortical fiber tract injuries may also cause aphasic disorders. These were termed conduction aphasias. Special attention has been paid lately to the aphasia produced by left thalamic lesions (2, 210, 244). It can be differentiated from conduction aphasia by the unimpaired ability to repeat spoken language.

4.11 Limbic System (Figs. 63 and 64)

The limbic system comprises cortical and subcortical portions (131). The cortical portions develop from archeocortex and periarcheocortex, which are phylogenetically older, and are pushed against the medial sides of both cerebral hemispheres by the development of the neocortex (290). These cortical parts form a margin around the corpus callosum and are called, therefore, "limbic". The archeocortex and periarcheocortex lie in front, above, and behind the corpus callosum and are divided into three corresponding subunits: the pre-, supra-, and retrocommissural cortices. The archeocortical portions form the inner edge of the margin, the periarcheocortical portions form the outer edge. The precommissural portion of the archeocortex includes the inner part of the subcallosal area; the supracommissural portion includes the supracallosal indusium griseum; and the retrocommissural portion includes the hippocampal formation. The outer ring around the corpus callosum is formed by the outer part of the subcallosal area, the part of the cingulate gyrus close to the corpus callosum and the parahippocampal gyrus (289). Electrophysiological stimulation of these regions leads to emotional reactions such as anger, fear, desire, sexual aggression, and the corresponding effects on the autonomic nervous system. Such observations led MacLean to name the limbic system the "visceral brain" (289).

The cortical limbic regions maintain afferent and efferent connections with certain subcortical structures. These subcortical structures – septum verum, preoptic area, mamillary body, other hypothalamic subnuclei, anterior nucleus of the thalamus, and limbic midbrain nuclei – are considered parts of the limbic system.

The subcallosal area and indusium griseum are relatively poorly developed in humans. The hippocampal formation, on the other hand, is larger in man than in apes (159, 289). It is located in the medial portion of the temporal lobe and consists of three parts: the hippocampus, dentate gyrus, and subiculum. During ontogenesis, the hippocampal formation is folded inward and comes to lie medial to the temporal horn of the lateral ventricle. It encloses the hippocampal sulcus in a C-shaped structure with two curved lips. The dentate gyrus lies in the upper limb of this structure. (The term dentate refers to the toothed appearance of the surface of the gyrus). The curved portion of the hippocampus extends into the lateral ventricle. The lower limb of the C is formed, for the most part, by the subiculum.

The hippocampal formation has afferent connections with the septum verum, hypothalamic subnuclei, parahippocampal gyrus, and the dopaminergic and serotoninergic centers of the brain stem (Chap. 4.12). A partially afferent pathway is a bundle of fibers, the fornix, which mainly carries efferent axons from the hippocampal formation. The fibers of the fornix form the alveus, a thin white layer on the ventricular surface of the hippocampus. They proceed as the fimbria of hippocampus and arch beneath the corpus callosum as the posterior pillar (crus) of the fornix. Under the splenium of the corpus callosum, where the right crus of the fornix meets the left crus, some fibers cross in the fornical commissure. Beneath the trunk of the corpus callosum the fornix descends toward the interventricular foramen (Monro). Here, the pathways separate into the two anterior pillars of fornix. These pillars skirt the interventricular foramen and continue, dorsally to the anterior commissure, in a caudal direction toward the hypothalamus. Directly above the anterior commissure, precommissural fibers extend to the septum verum, gyrus rectus, and frontal cortex. Below the anterior commissure, fiber bundles reach the nuclei of the stria terminalis and the anterior nucleus of the thalamus. The main bundle of the fornix projects into the hypothalamus, where the majority of the fibers terminate in the mamillary body.

The mamillothalamic tract (Vicq d'Azyr's bundle) projects from the mamillary body to the anterior nucleus of the thalamus. Fiber pathways return via the cingulum to the hippocampal formation. This circuit (hippocampal formation → mamillary body → anterior nucleus of the thalamus → cingulate gyrus and cingulum → hippocampal formation) is known as Papez circuit (206). Connections radiate from here into the frontal cortex, cingulate gyrus, and parahippocampal gyrus. These neuronal connections are

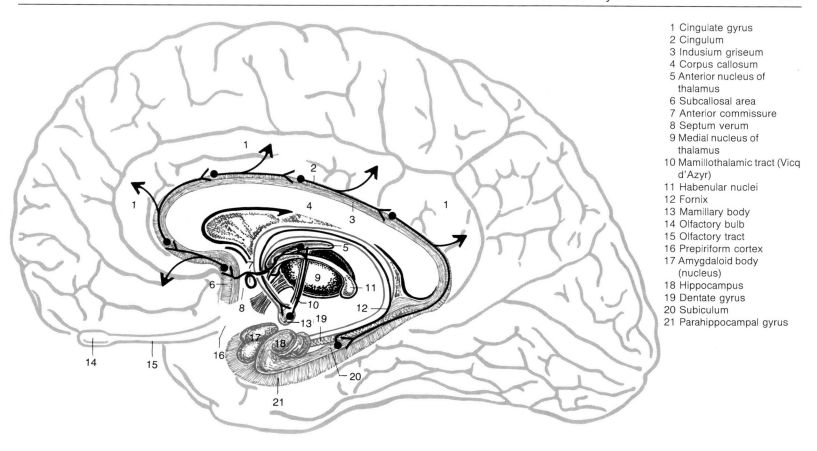

Fig. 63 Medial view of the limbic and olfactory systems. The wall of the third ventricle has been omitted revealing Papez circuit, mamillothalamic tract (Vicq d'Azyr), and anterior nucleus of the thalamus. According to (206, 289).

most likely to be affected when a bilateral lesion of the hippocampal formation, the fornices, or the mamillary bodies causes a dramatic loss of recent memory (132, 250).

The amygdaloid body is a complex of several nuclei and a cortical area. It is located in a medial position at the tip of the temporal horn of the lateral ventricle and belongs partly to the olfactory centers (Chap. 4.7) and partly to the limbic system. The amygdaloid body has afferent connections with the olfactory bulb, hypothalamic nuclei, brain stem, and cortical regions of the telencephalon. The main efferent pathways are the stria terminalis and the ventral amygdalofugal fibers. The stria terminalis arches between the caudate nucleus and the thalamus and projects into the septum verum, hypothalamic nuclei, reticular formation, and into isolated telencephalic regions.

The septum verum, namely the septal nuclei and precommissural septum, plays a central role among the subcortical nuclear areas of the limbic system

mentioned earlier. The medial forebrain bundle connects the septum verum with other centers. This connection is twofold as far as the midbrain, namely septomesencephalic and mesencephaloseptic. These centers are the preoptic regions of the hypothalamus, lateral and medial hypothalamic nuclei, and limbic nuclear areas of the midbrain. The latter include a ventral region of the mesencephalic tegmentum, the interpeduncular nucleus, as well as the dorsal raphe nucleus, the superior central nucleus (Bechterew), and the dorsal tegmental nucleus (Gudden). The mamillotegmental tract connects the mamillary body with the tegmentum of the midbrain. A further connection exists between the hypothalamic centers and the medulla oblongata via the dorsal longitudinal fasciculus (Schütz). The striae medullares thalami bypass the hypothalamus and project from septum verum and hypothalamic regions to the habenular nuclei. The habenulointerpeduncular tract continues from the habenular nuclei to the interpeduncular nucleus.

1 Periarcheocortex
  (retrocommissural)
2 Amygdaloid body (nu-
  cleus) (partially belong-
  ing to the limbic system)
3 Hippocampal formation
4 Subcallosal area
5 Mamillary body (within the
  slice)
6 Uncus of parahippocampal
  gyrus
7 Parahippocampal gyrus
8 Periarcheocortex in the
  cingulate gyrus
9 Septum verum
10 Fornix

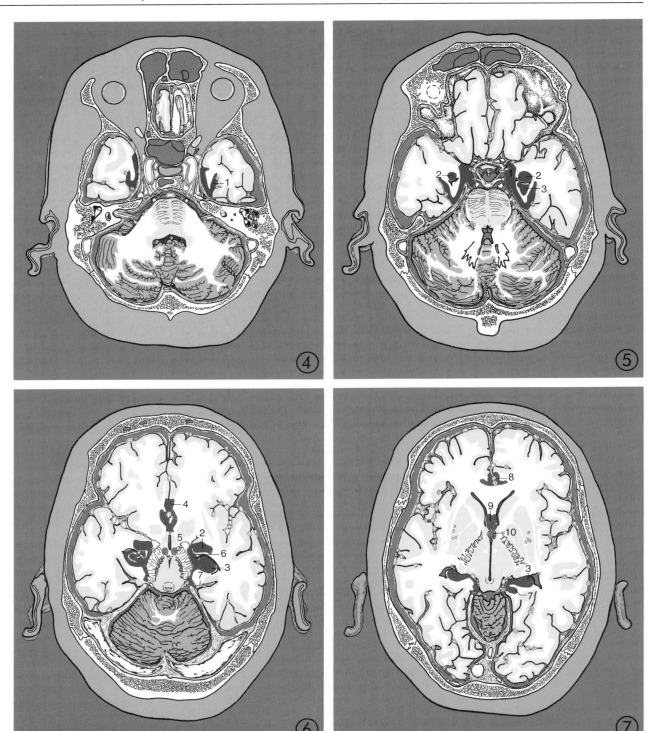

Fig. 64 Serial illustrations of the cortical areas and the most important nuclear regions of the limbic system including the fornix and the mamillary body. The encircled number indicates the number of the respective slice (see Figs. 1a, 2, 3, 4).

1 Periarcheocortex
  (retrocommissural)
3 Hippocampal formation
8 Periarcheocortex in the
  cingulate gyrus
10 Fornix

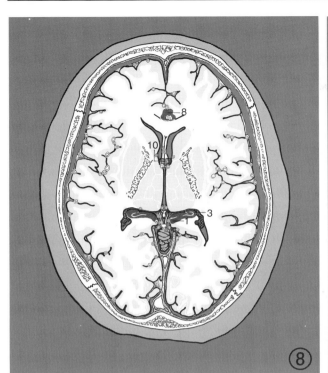

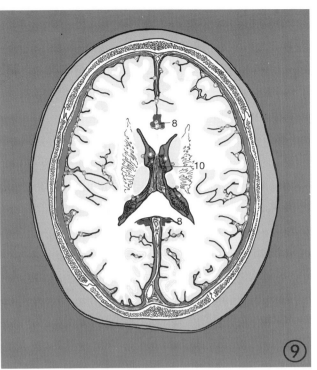

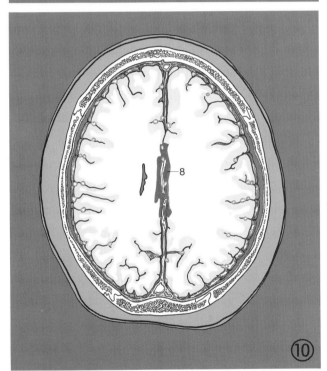

4.12 Monoaminergic Systems

Cell bodies and axons of the monoaminergic neurons utilize one of three biogenic amines as transmitter substance: dopamine, noradrenaline, or serotonin. These substances have a low molecular weight and are derived from the amino acids tyrosine (dopamine and noradrenaline) or tryptophan (serotonin). As a result of their low molecular weight, all three of these transmitter substances diffuse easily out of the nerve cells and axons post mortem. Conventional histological techniques are not successful in determining the production and storage locations of these substances in living cells.

In 1962 the discovery of the dopaminergic, noradrenergic, and serotoninergic neurons was made possible technically by first freezing the living nerve cells and then drying them prior to examination with fluorescent microscopy. Histochemical techniques were successful in demonstrating a green fluorescence for dopamine and noradrenaline and a yellow fluorescence for serotonin (67). Today, the more sensitive immunofluorescent methods enable more accurate proof of monoaminergic neurons. The noradrenergic and dopaminergic nerve cells are labelled from A1 to A15, the serotoninergic cells from B1 to B9. The numbers are given in an ascending order along the brain stem, in other words, from caudal to cranial.

The mapping of the monoaminergic cell groups and pathways is the subject of continuing investigation. Results, that have been derived from rats and a select number of primate brains, must be extrapolated to the human brain. The dopaminergic, nigrostriate system is undoubtedly of importance in Parkinson's disease. Monoaminergic systems are the probable reaction sites of antidepressants and neuroleptics (186). Therefore, current knowledge of monoaminergic systems, although still incomplete, is of great interest for medicine today.

The presently limited geometric resolution of computed tomography does not provide the basis for an exact location of the monoaminergic systems in CT scans. For this reason, a more general identification of the portions of the brain, that house the monoaminergic systems, must suffice. The positions of the medulla oblongata, pons, cerebellum, midbrain, diencephalon, and telencephalon are illustrated in a medial view (Fig. 34) and in serial illustrations (Fig. 35).

4.12.1 Dopaminergic Systems

Dopamine producing nerve cells are located in the midbrain, diencephalon, and telencephalon. The largest and most obvious group of dopaminergic nerve cells is the pars compacta of the substantia nigra (A9) (Figs. 10b.29, 56.10, 58.2). The axons of these nerve cells form a large ascending pathway that extends through the lateral part of the hypothalamus, traverses the internal capsule, and projects into the striatum (caudate nucleus and putamen). The small cell group A8 from the mesencephalic reticular formation together with the cell group A9 forms the nigrostriatal system. Based on its synaptic connections, the substantia nigra is considered part of the basal ganglia (Chap. 4.8.2).

A second dopaminergic system extends from the mesencephalic cell group A10 to parts of the limbic system and is referred to as the mesolimbic dopaminergic system. Drugs affecting this system are supposed to elicit psychic effects (186). The cell group A10 lies as a ventral cap on the interpeduncular nucleus in the mesencephalic tegmentum. The axons project via the medial forebrain bundle into the following limbic structures: the bed nucleus of the stria terminalis, olfactory tubercle, nucleus accumbens, lateral septal nucleus, and several portions of the frontal, cingulate, and entorhinal cortices.

A third dopaminergic system, the tuberoinfundibular system, is located in the diencephalon. The cell group A12 lies in the tuber cinereum and projects to the median eminence. The system has a neuroendocrine function. The other diencephalic cell groups A11, A13, A14, and their projections are also located within the hypothalamus. A small cell group, A15, is scattered throughout the olfactory bulb and is the only dopaminergic group of neurons located in the telencephalon. The use of dopamine substitutes, which prove beneficial in the treatment of conditions such as Parkinson's disease (Chap. 4.8.2), has illuminated the clinical significance of dopamine deficiency, especially in the substantia nigra (84, 185, 193, 217).

4.12.2 Noradrenergic Systems

The noradrenergic nerve cells are located in the tegmentum of the medulla oblongata and pons. Although the cell groups A1 to A7 have been described primarily in rats (49, 50), similar arrangements may also be found in primates (70, 85, 126, 127, 186, 194, 208). The fibers projecting from these nerve cells either ascend toward the midbrain or descend in a spinal direction. In addition, noradrenergic nerve cells are connected with the cerebellum. The noradrenergic fibers are branched wider than the dopaminergic fibers. The proximity of the noradrenergic fibers to cerebral arterioles and capillaries is conspicuous. The noradrenergic fibers, therefore, probably play a role in the regulation of cerebral blood flow (102, 236).

The largest noradrenergic cell group A6 lies in the locus ceruleus and contains almost half of all noradrenergic cells (294). In adults, the locus ceruleus contains melanin-pigmented nerve cells. They form a bluish-black stripe. It is approximately 1 cm long and runs along the floor of the fourth ventricle in the pontine region (Figs. 9b.20 and 10b.34) reaching as far as the tectum of the midbrain. The dorsal noradrenergic bundle originates in this A6 group. The bundle extends via the tegmentum of the midbrain in a ventrolateral position to the periaqueductal gray matter, enters the hypothalamus, and runs toward the septal region and the cingulum. The dorsal noradrenergic bundle is connected with the following structures:

● Dorsal raphe nuclei and superior and inferior colliculi in the mesencephalon
● Anterior nucleus of the thalamus and medial and lateral geniculate bodies in the diencephalon
● Amygdaloid body, hippocampal formation, entire neocortex, and the cingulate, retrosplenial, and entorhinal cortices in the telencephalon.

Additional fibers of the group A6 project into the cerebellum via the superior cerebellar peduncle. Descending fibers from the locus ceruleus are accompanied by fibers from the neighboring cell group A7, and supply the dorsal nucleus of the vagus nerve, the inferior olivary nucleus, and the spinal cord. The ventrolateral ceruleospinal pathway shares noradrenergic fibers with the anterior and posterior horns of the spinal cord (209). As a whole, the few noradrenergic cells of the locus ceruleus have an immense field of projection, reaching into the forebrain, cerebellum, brain stem, and spinal cord.

The cell groups A1 and A2 lie in the medulla oblongata and, together with the pontine cell groups A5 and A7, form the ascending ventral noradrenergic system. In the mesencephalon these neurons project into the periaqueductal gray matter and the reticular formation. In the diencephalon they project into the entire hypothalamus and in the telencephalon into the olfactory bulb. Additionally, bulbospinal fibers descend from these cell groups (A1, A2, A5, A7) into the spinal cord.

4.12.3 Serotoninergic Systems

The serotoninergic nerve cells B1 to B9 are located in the medulla oblongata, pons, and midbrain (nomenclature according to 49, 50). The majority of these cell groups occupy the midline of the brain stem ("suture-zone" = "raphe") and are, therefore, referred to as the raphe nuclei. The raphe nuclei B1 (nucleus raphe pallidus) and B2 (nucleus raphe obscurus) lie in the medulla oblongata. B3 (nucleus raphe magnus) is located at the border between the medulla oblongata and pons. B5 (nucleus raphe pontis) lies in the pons and B7 (nucleus raphe dorsalis) in the midbrain. The cell groups B6 and B8 (superior central nucleus (Bechterew)) are located in the tegmentum of the pons and midbrain.

Like the noradrenergic system, the serotoninergic system has both ascending and descending projections. The principal serotoninergic projections are directed into the limbic system, the reticular formation, and the spinal cord. A close connection also exists with the locus ceruleus, the largest noradrenergic center. The large ascending ventral pathway originates in the cell groups B6, B8, and B7. It extends ventrally through the tegmentum of the midbrain and laterally through the hypothalamus before branching into the pathways of the fornix and cingulum. The cell groups B6, B8, and B7 are synaptically connected with the following structures:

● Interpeduncular nucleus and substantia nigra in the mesencephalon
● Habenular nuclei, small thalamic subnuclei, and hypothalamic nuclei in the diencephalon
● Septal nuclei and olfactory bulb in the telencephalon.

Extensive projections to further limbic regions, such as the hippocampus, the subiculum, and the cingulate and entorhinal cortices also exist. There are, as well, connections with the striatum and the frontal neocortex. The shorter, dorsal ascending pathway connects cell groups B3, B5, and B7 via the dorsal longitudinal fasciculus (Schütz) with the mesencephalic periaqueductal gray matter and the posterior hypothalamic area. In addition, serotoninergic fibers project into the cerebellum (B6 and B7) and spinal cord (B1 to B3). Numerous connections also exist with the reticular formation. These findings correspond well to observations on serotoninergic sleep mechanisms.

5 References

1 Adams, R.D., Victor, M.: Principles of neurology. 2nd ed. New York: McGraw Hill 1981

2 Alexander, M.P., Lo Verme, St.R.: Aphasia after left hemispheric intracerebral hemorrhage. Neurology 30 (1980) 1193–1202

3 Alfidi, R.J., Haaga, J.R., El Yousef, S.J., Bryan, P.J., Fletcher, B.D., Li Puma, J.P., Morrison, St.C., Kaufman, B., Richey, J.B, Hinshaw, W.S., Kramer, D.M., Yeung, H.N., Cohen, A.M., Butler, H.E., Ament, A.E., Lieberman, J.M.: Preliminary experimental results in humans and animals with a superconducting, whole-body, nuclear magnetic resonance scanner. Radiology 143 (1982) 175–181

4 Alpers, B.J., Berry, R.G.: Circle of Willis in cerebral vascular disorders. Arch. Neurol. 8 (1963) 398–402

5 Ambrose, J.: Computerized transverse axial scanning (tomography). Part 2: Clinical application. Brit. J. Radiol. 46 (1973) 1023–1047

6 Andres, K.H., Düring, M. von: General methods for characterization of brain regions. In: Heym, Ch., Forssmann, W.-G.: Techniques in neuroanatomical research. Berlin, Heidelberg, New York: Springer 1981 100–108

7 Angevine, J.B. (Jr.), Mancall, E.L., Yakovlev, P.I.: The human cerebellum. An atlas of cross topography in serial sections. Boston: Little and Brown 1961

8 Arey, L.B.: Developmental anatomy. A textbook and laboratory manual of embryology. Philadelphia, London: Saunders 1965

9 Armond, St.J. de, Fusco, M.M., Dewey, M.M.: Structure of the human brain. A photographic atlas. New York: Oxford University Press 1976

10 Baumgartner, G.: Funktion und Symptomatik einzelner Hirnregionen. In: Hopf, H.Ch., Poeck, K., Schliack, H. (Eds.): Neurologie in Praxis und Klinik. Vol. I. Stuttgart: Thieme 1983 1.77–1.112

11 Beevor, C.E.: On the distribution of the different arteries supplying the human brain. Phil. Trans. B 200 (1909) 1–55

12 Benjamin, R.M., Burton, H.: Projection of taste nerve afferents to anterior opercular-insular cortex in squirrel monkey (Saimiri sciureus). Brain Res. 7 (1968) 221–231

13 Benninghoff, A., Goerttler, K., Ferner, H, Staubesand, J. (Eds.): Lehrbuch der Anatomie des Menschen. Vol. 3: Nervensystem, Haut und Sinnesorgane. München, Wien, Baltimore: Urban und Schwarzenberg 1979

14 Benson, D.F.: Neurological correlates of aphasia and apraxia. In: Matthews, W.B., Glaser, G.H. (Eds.). Recent advances in clinical neurology. Edinburgh, London, New York: Livingstone 1978 163–175

15 Berman, St.A., Hayman, L.A., Hinck, V.C.: Correlation of CT cerebral vascular territories with function: I. Anterior cerebral artery. Amer. J. Roentgenol. 135 (1980) 253–257

16 Berman, St.A., Hayman, L.A., Hinck, V.C.: Correlation of CT cerebral vascular territories with function: III. Middle cerebral artery. Amer. J. Roentgenol. 142 (1984) 1035–1040

17 Berns, T.F., Daniels, D.L., Williams, A.L., Haughton, V.M.: Mesencephalic anatomy: Demonstration by computed tomography. Amer. J. Neuroradiol. 2 (1981) 65–67

18 Bierny, J.-P., Komar, N.N.: The sylvian cistern on computed tomography scanning. J. Comput. assist. Tomogr. 1 (1977) 227–230

19 Biersack, H.J., Knopp, R., Winkler, C.: Emissionscomputertomographie. Therapiewoche 31 (1981) 6067–6079

20 Bilaniuk, L.T., Zimmerman, R.A., Wehrli, F.W., Goldberg, H.I., Grossman, R.I., Bottomley, P.A., Edelstein, W.A., Glover, G.H., MacFall, J.R., Redington, R.W., Kressel, H.Y.: Cerebral magnetic resonance: Comparison of high and low field strength imaging. Radiology 153 (1984) 409–414

21 Birg, W., Mundinger, F.: Direct target point determination for stereotactic brain operations from CT data and the calculation of setting parameters for polar-coordinate stereotactic devices. Appl. Neurophysiol. 45 (1982) 387–395

22 Bliesener, J.A.: Intrakranielle Veränderungen im Säuglings- und frühen Kindesalter. Mschr. Kinderheilk. 129 (1981) 200–215

23 Bliesener, J.A., Sperlich, D.: Der Stellenwert der Ultraschalluntersuchung des Schädels im frühen Kindesalter. Radiologe 21 (1981) 527–537

24 Blunk, R., Bleser, R. de, Willmes, K., Zeumer, H.: A refined method to relate morphological and functional aspects of aphasia. Europ. Neurol. 20 (1981) 69–79

25 Bo, W.J., Meschan, I., Krueger, W.A.: Basic atlas of cross-sectional anatomy. Philadelphia, London, Toronto: Saunders 1980

26 Bodechtel, G.: Differentialdiagnose neurologischer Krankheitsbilder. 4th ed. Stuttgart: Thieme 1984

27 Bowsher, D.: Diencephalic projections from the midbrain reticular formation. Brain Res. 95 (1975) 211–220

28 Braak, H.: Architectonics of the human telencephalic cortex. Berlin, Heidelberg, New York: Springer 1980

29 Brant-Zawadzki, M., Davis, P.L., Crooks, L.E., Mills, C.M., Norman, D., Newton, Th.H., Sheldon, P., Kaufman, L.: NMR demonstration of cerebral abnormalities: Comparison with CT. Amer. J. Roentgenol. 140 (1983) 847–854

30 Brassow, F., Baumann, K.: Volume of brain ventricles in man determined by computer tomography. Neuroradiology 16 (1978) 187–189

31 Brietze, K.-H., Krysewski, M.: Qualitative und quantitative Untersuchung des Nucl. motorius n. trigemini an ontogenetischen Reihen männlicher SPF-Katzen und Tupaia belangeri. J. Hirnforsch. 20 (1979) 507–527

32 Brodal, A.: Anatomy of the vestibular nuclei and their connections. In: Autrum, H., Jung, R., Loewenstein, W.R., Mackay, D.M., Teuber, H. (Eds.): Handbook of sensory physiology. Vol. VI: Vestibular system, part 1. Berlin, Heidelberg, New York: Springer 1974 239–352

33 Brodal, A.: Neurological anatomy in relation to clinical medicine. New York, Oxford: Oxford University Press 1981

34 Broser, F.: Topische und klinische Diagnostik neurologischer Krankheiten. München, Wien, Baltimore: Urban und Schwarzenberg 1981

35 Brown, B.St.J., Tissington Tatlow, W.F.: Radiographic studies of the vertebral arteries in cadavers, effects of position and traction on the head. Radiology 81 (1963) 80–88

36 Brust, J.C.M.: Stroke. Diagnostic, anatomical, and physiological considerations. In: Kandel, E.R., Schwartz, J.H. (Eds.): Principles of neural science. New York: Elsevier Science Publishing 1983 667–679

37 Bucher, O.: Cytologie, Histologie und mikroskopische Anatomie des Menschen. Bern, Stuttgart, Wien: Huber 1980

38 Buren, J.M. van, Borke, R.C.: Variations and connections of the human thalamus. 2 Vols. Berlin, Heidelberg, New York: Springer 1972

39 Burian, K., Fanta, H., Reisner, H.: Neurootologie. Stuttgart, New York: Thieme 1980

40 Burton, H., Benjamin, R.M.: Central projections of the gustatory system. In: Autrum, H., Jung, R., Loewenstein, W.R., Mackay, D.M., Teuber, H.L. (Eds.): Handbook of sensory physiology. Vol. IV: Chemical senses, part 2. Berlin, Heidelberg, New York: Springer 1971 148–164

41 Carpenter, M.B., Sutin, J.: Human neuroanatomy. 8th ed. Baltimore: Williams and Wilkens 1983

42 Carpenter, M.B.: Anatomy and physiology of the basal ganglia. In: Schaltenbrand, G., Walker, A.E. (Eds.): Stereotaxy of the human brain. 2nd ed. Stuttgart, New York: Thieme 1982 233–268

43 Carter, B.L., Morehead, J., Wolpert, S.M., Hammerschlag, St.B., Griffiths, H.J., Kahn, P.C.: Cross-sectional anatomy. Computed tomography and ultrasound correlation. New York: Appleton-Century-Crofts 1977

44 Chynn, K.-Y., Finby, N.: Manual of cranial computerized tomography. Basel: Karger 1982

45 Citrin, C.M., Alper, M.G.: Computed tomography of the visual pathways. Comput. Tomogr. 3 (1979) 305–331

46 Citrin, C.M., Alper, M.G.: Computed tomography of the visual pathways. Int. Ophthalmol. Clin. 22 (1982) 155–180

47 Clar, H.-E., Bock, W.J., Grote, W., Löhr, E.: Atlas der Enzephalotomographie. Stuttgart: Thieme 1976

48 Crosby, E.C., Humphrey, T., Lauer, E.W.: Correlative anatomy of the nervous system. New York: Macmillan 1962

49 Dahlström, A., Fuxe, K.: Evidence for the existence of monoamine-containing neurons in the central nervous system. I. Demonstration of monoamines in the cell bodies of brain stem neurons. Acta physiol. scand. 62, Suppl. 232 (1964) 1–55

50 Dahlström, A., Fuxe, K.: Evidence for the existence of monoamine neurons in the central nervous system. II. Experimentally induced changes in the intraneuronal amine levels of bulbospinal neuron systems. Acta physiol. scand. 64, Suppl. 247 (1965) 1–36

51 Damasio, H.: A computed tomographic guide to the identification of cerebral vascular territories. Arch. Neurol. 40 (1983) 138–142

52 Daniels, D.L., Williams, A.L., Haughton, V.M.: Computed tomography of the medulla. Radiology 145 (1982) 63–69

53 Darian-Smith, I.: The trigeminal system. In: Autrum, H., Jung, R., Loewenstein, W.R., Mackay, D.M., Teuber, H.L. (Eds.): Handbook of sensory physiology. Vol. II: Somatosensory system. Berlin, Heidelberg, New York: Springer 1973 271–314

54 Dejerine, J.: Anatomie des centres nerveux. Tome I/II. Paris: Rueff 1895–1901

55 Dejong, R.N.: The neurologic examination. New York, Evanston, London: Harper and Row 1979

56 Dekaban, A.S.: Tables of cranial and orbital measurements, cranial volume, and derived indexes in males and females. From 7 days to 20 years of age. Ann. Neurol. 2 (1977) 485–491

57 Denny-Brown, D.: Relations and functions of the pyramidal tract. In: Schaltenbrand, G., Walker, A.E. (Eds.): Stereotaxy of the human brain, 2nd ed. Stuttgart, New York: Thieme 1982 131–139

58 Dewulf, A.: Anatomy of the normal human thalamus. Amsterdam: Elsevier 1971

59 Diepen, R.: Der Hypothalamus. In: Möllendorff, W. von, Bargmann, W., Oksche, A., Vollrath, L. (Eds.): Handbuch der mikroskopischen Anatomie des Menschen. Vol. 4: Nervensystem, part 7. Berlin, Heidelberg, New York: Springer 1962

60 Droege, R.T., Wiener, St.N., Rzeszotarski, M.S.: A strategy for magnetic resonance imaging of the head: Results of a semi-empirical model. Part I. Radiology 153 (1984) 419–424

61 Droege, R.T., Wiener, St.N., Rzeszotarski, M.S.: A strategy for magnetic resonance imaging of the head: Results of a semi-empirical model. Part II. Radiology 153 (1984) 425–433

62 Duus, P.: Topical diagnosis in neurology. Anatomy, physiology, signs, symptoms. Stuttgart, New York: Thieme-Stratton 1983

63 Eccles, J.C., Ito, M., Szentagothai, J.: The cerebellum as a neuronal machine. Berlin, Heidelberg, New York: Springer 1967

64 Economo, C. von, Koskinas, G.N.: Die Cytoarchitektonik der Hirnrinde des erwachsenen Menschen. Text and atlas. Wien, Berlin: Springer 1925

65 Ell, P.J., Deacon, J.M., Jarritt, H.: Atlas of computerized emission tomography. Edinburgh, London, New York: Churchill Livingstone 1980

66 Englander, R.N., Netsky, M.G., Adelman, L.S.: Location of human pyramidal tract in the internal capsule: Anatomic evidence. Neurology 25 (1975) 823–826

67 Falck, B., Hillarp, N.-A., Thieme, G., Torp, A.: Fluorescence of catecholamines and related compounds condensed with formaldehyde. J. Histochem. Cytochem. 10 (1962) 348–354

68 Farruggia, S., Babcock, D.S.: The cavum septi pellucidi: Its appearance and incidence with cranial ultrasonography in infancy. Radiology 139 (1981) 147–150

69 Felix, R., Ramm, B.: Das Röntgenbild, 2nd ed. Stuttgart: Thieme 1982

70 Felten, D.L., Laties, A.M., Carpenter, M.B.: Monoamine-containing cell bodies in the squirrel monkey brain. Amer. J. Anat. 139 (1974) 153–166

71 Feneis, H.: Pocket atlas of human anatomy. Based on the international nomenclature. Stuttgart, New York: Thieme 1985

72 Ferner, H., Kautzky, R.: Angewandte Anatomie des Gehirns und seiner Hüllen. In: Krenkel, W., Olivecrona, H., Tönnis, W. (Eds.): Handbuch der Neurochirurgie. Vol. I: Grundlagen, part 1: Angewandte Anatomie, Physiologie und Pathophysiologie. Berlin, Göttingen, Heidelberg: Springer 1959

73 Fischer, T., Schietzel, M.: Bildgebende Verfahren. Medizintechnik 104 (1984) 99–102

74 FitzGerald, M.J.T.: Neuroanatomy basic and applied. London, Philadelphia, Toronto: Baillière Tindall 1985

75 Foerster, O.: Motorische Felder und Bahnen. Sensible corticale Felder. In: Bumke, O., Foerster, O. (Eds.): Handbuch der Neurologie. Vol. VI. Berlin: Springer 1936 1–488

76 Forssmann, W.G., Heym, C.: Neuroanatomie. Berlin, Heidelberg, New York: Springer 1985

77 Fredrickson, J.M., Kornhuber, H.H., Schwarz, D.W.F.: Cortical projections of the vestibular nerve. In: Autrum, H., Jung, R., Loewenstein, W.R., Mackay, D.W., Teuber, H.L. (Eds.): Handbook of sensory physiology. Vol. VI: Vestibular system, part I: Basic mechanisms. Berlin, Heidelberg, New York: Springer 1974 565–582

78 Fritsch, R., Hitzig, E.: Über die elektrische Erregbarkeit des Großhirns. Arch. Anat. Physiol. u. wissenschaftl. Med. 37 (1870) 300–332

79 Froriep, A.: Die Lagebeziehungen zwischen Großhirn und Schädeldach. Leipzig: Veit 1897

80 Gado, M., Hanaway, J., Frank, R.: Functional anatomy of the cerebral cortex by computed tomography. J. Comput. assist. Tomogr. 3 (1979) 1–19

81 Gambarelli, J., Guérinel, G., Chevrot, L., Mattèi, M.: Computerized axial tomography. Berlin, Heidelberg, New York: Springer 1977

82 Gänshirt, H.: Zerebrale Zirkulationsstörungen. In: Hopf, H.Ch., Poeck, K., Schliack, H. (Eds.): Neurologie in Praxis und Klinik. Vol. I. Stuttgart, New York: Thieme 1983 2.1–2.83

83 Ganssen, A., Loeffler, W., Oppelt, A., Schmidt, F.: Kernspin-Tomographie. Computertomographie 1 (1981) 10–18

84 Garnett, E.S., Nahmias, C., Firnau, G.: Central dopaminergic pathways in hemiparkinsonism examined by positron emission tomography. Can. J. Neurol. Sci. 11 (1984) 174–179

85 Garver, D.L., Sladek, J.R. (Jr.): Monoamine distribution in primate brain. I. Catecholamine-containing perikarya in the brain stem of Macaca speciosa. J. comp. Neurol. 159 (1975) 289–304

86 Geschwind, N.: Specializations of the human brain. Scientific American 241 (1979) 180–199

87 Glaser, J.S.: Neuro-ophthalmology. Hagerstown/Maryland: Harper and Row 1978

88 Gluhbegovic, N., Williams, T.H.: The human brain: A photographic guide. Hagerstown/Maryland: Harper and Row 1980

89 Goldammer, E. von: Physikalische Grundlagen der magnetischen Kernspintomographie. Medizintechnik 104 (1984) 84–98

90 Gudden, F.: Bildgebende Systeme heute und morgen. Electromedica 49 (1981) 64–67

91 Haaga, J.R., Alfidi, R.J. (Eds.): Computed tomography of the whole body. Saint Louis: Mosby 1983

92 Habermehl, A., Graul, E.H.: Kernspinresonanz-Tomographie. Physikalisch-technische Grundlagen, klinische Anwendungen und Perspektiven. Dtsch. Ärztebl. 79 (1982) 17–29

93 Hacker, H., Artmann, H.: The calculation of CSF spaces in CT. Neuroradiology 16 (1978) 190–192

94 Hacker, H., Kühner, G.: Die Brückenvenen. Radiologe 12 (1972) 45–48

95 Hamilton, W.J., Mossman, H.W.: Human embryology. 4th ed. Baltimore: Williams and Wilkins 1972

96 Hammock, M.K., Milhorat, Th.H.: Cranial computed tomography in infancy and childhood. Baltimore: Williams and Wilkins 1981

97 Hanaway, J., Scott, W.R., Strother, C.M.: Atlas of the human brain and the orbit for computed tomography. St. Louis: Green 1980

98 Hanaway, J., Young, R.R.: Localization of the pyramidal tract in the internal capsule of man. J. Neurol. Sci. 34 (1977) 63–70

99 Hanaway, J., Young, R., Netsky, M., Adelman, L.: Localization of the pyramidal tract in the internal capsule. Neurology 31 (1981) 365–367

100 Hardy, T.L., Bertrand, G., Thompson, C.J.: The position and organization of motor fibers in the internal capsule found during stereotactic surgery. Appl. Neurophysiol. 42 (1979) 160–170

101 Harrison, J.M., Howe, M.E.: Anatomy of the afferent auditory nervous system of mammals. In: Autrum, H., Jung, R., Loewenstein, W.R., Mackay, D.W., Teuber, H.L. (Eds.): Handbook of sensory physiology. Vol. V: Auditory system, part 1. Berlin, Heidelberg, New York: Springer 1974 283–336

102 Hartman, B.K.: The innervation of cerebral blood vessels by central noradrenergic neurons. In: Usdin, E., Snyder, S.H. (Eds.): Frontiers in catecholamine research. Oxford: Pergamon Press 1973 91–96

103 Hartwig, H.G., Wahren, W.: Anatomy of the hypothalamus. In: Schaltenbrand, G., Walker, A.E. (Eds.): Stereotaxy of the human brain, 2nd ed. Stuttgart, New York: Thieme 1982 87–106

104 Hassler, R.: Anatomy of the thalamus. In: Schaltenbrand, G., Bailey, P. (Eds.): Introduction to stereotaxis, with an atlas of the human brain. Vol. I. New York: Grune and Stratton 1959 230–290

105 Hassler, R., Mundinger, F., Riechert, T.: Stereotaxis in Parkinson Syndrome. Berlin, Heidelberg, New York: Springer 1979

106 Hassler, R.: Neuronale Grundlagen der spastischen Tonussteigerung. In: Bauer, H.J., Koella, W.P., Struppler, A. (Eds.): Therapie der Spastik. München: Verlag für angewandte Wissenschaften 1981

107 Hassler, R.: Architectonic organization of the thalamic nuclei. In: Schaltenbrand, G., Walker, A.E. (Eds.): Stereotaxy of the human brain, 2nd ed. Stuttgart, New York: Thieme 1982 140–180

108 Haug, H.: The significance of quantitative stereologic experimental procedures in pathology. Path. Res. Pract. 166 (1980) 144–164

109 Haverling, M.: The tortuous basilar artery. Acta radiol. Diagn. 15 (1974) 241–249

110 Hayman, L.A., Berman, S.A., Hinck, V.C.: Correlation of CT cerebral vascular territories with function. II. Posterior cerebral artery. Amer. J. Radiol. 137 (1981) 13–19

111 Hécaen, H.: Cortical localization of function. In: Schaltenbrand, G., Walker, A.E. (Eds.): Stereotaxy of the human brain, 2nd ed. Stuttgart, New York: Thieme 1982 293–305

112 Heidary, A., Tomasch, J.: Neuron numbers and perikaryon areas in the human cerebellar nuclei. Acta anat. (Basel) 74 (1969) 290–296

113 Heimer, L.: The human brain and spinal cord. Functional neuroanatomy and dissection guide. New York, Berlin, Heidelberg, Tokyo: Springer 1983

114 Heimer, L., Roards, M.J. (Eds.): Neuroanatomical tract-tracing methods. New York: Plenum 1981

115 Heiss, W.D., Phelps, M.E.: Positron emission tomography of the brain. Berlin, Heidelberg, New York: Springer 1983

116 Heller, M., Jend, H.-H., Grabbe, E., Hambüchen, K.: Seriencomputertomographie. Electromedica 49 (1981) 68–73

117 Henry, J.M.: Anatomy of the brainstem. In: Schaltenbrand, G., Walker, A.E. (Eds.): Stereotaxy of the human brain, 2nd ed. Stuttgart, New York: Thieme 1982 37–59

118 Heym, C., Forssmann, W.-G. (Eds.): Techniques in neuroanatomical research. Berlin, Heidelberg, New York: Springer 1981

119 Hilal, S.K., Trokel, St.L.: Computerized tomography of the orbit using thin sections. Semin. Roentgenol. 12 (1977) 137–147

120 Hilal, S.K., Trokel, St.L., Coleman, D.J.: High resolution computerized tomography and B-scan ultrasonography of the orbits. Trans. Amer. Acad. Ophthal. Otolaryng. 81 (1976) 607–617

121 Hiller, D., Ermert, H.: Computer-Tomographie mit Ultraschall. Biomed. Technik 26 (1981) 64–65

122 Hobson, J.A., Brazier, M.A.B. (Eds.): The reticular formation revisited. New York: Raven 1980

123 Holman, B.L., Hill, T.C., Magistretti, P.L.: Brain imaging with emission computed tomography and radiolabeled amines. Invest. Radiol. 17 (1982) 206–215

124 Hopf, H.Ch., Poeck, K., Schliack, H. (Eds.): Neurologie in Praxis und Klinik. 3 Vols. Stuttgart: Thieme
Vol. 1: Zerebrale und spinale Lokalisationslehre, zerebrale und spinale Zirkulationsstörungen, traumatische Schädigung des zentralen Nervensystems, Kopf- und Gesichtsschmerzen, Koma, extrapyramidale Krankheiten, Mißbildungen und frühkindliche Schäden des Nervensystems einschließlich Hydrozephalus. 1983
Vol. 2: Muskelkrankheiten, Polyneuropathien, Intoxikationen, entzündliche Erkrankungen des ZNS, multiple Sklerose, Epilepsie, nichtepileptische Anfälle. 1981
Vol. 3: Peripheres Nervensystem, heredodegenerative Krankheiten, stoffwechselbedingte und dystrophische Krankheitsprozesse, Phakomatosen, neurokutane Syndrome, raumfordernde Prozesse, Gefäßtumoren, Skelettsystem, psychogene Symptomatik. 1985

125 Hounsfield, G.N.: Computerized transverse axial scanning (tomography). Part I: Description of system. Brit. J. Radiol. 46 (1973) 1016–1022

126 Hubbard, J.E., Carlo, V. di: Fluorescence histochemistry of monoamine-containing cell bodies in the brain stem of the squirrel monkey (Saimiri sciureus). II. Catecholamine-containing groups. J. comp. Neurol. 153 (1974) 369–384

127 Hubbard, J.E., Carlo, V. di: Fluorescence histochemistry of monoamine-containing cell bodies in the brain stem of the squirrel monkey (Saimiri sciureus). III. Serotonin-containing groups. J. comp. Neurol. 153 (1974) 385–398

128 Huber, P., Krayenbühl, H., Yasargil, M.G.: Cerebral angiography. Stuttgart, New York: Thieme-Stratton 1982

129 Hübner, K.F., Purvis, J.T., Mahaley, S.M. (Jr.), Robertson, J.T., Rogers, S., Gibbs, W.D., King, P., Partain, C.L.: Brain tumor imaging by positron emission computed tomography using C-labeled amino acids. J. Comput. assist. Tomogr. 6 (1982) 544–550

130 International Anatomical Nomenclature Committee Nomina Anatomica, 5th ed. Approved by the eleventh international congress of anatomists at Mexico City 1980. Baltimore: Williams and Wilkins 1983

131 Isaacson, R.L.: The limbic system. 2nd ed. New York, London: Plenum 1982

132 Iversen, S.D.: Do hippocampal lesions produce amnesia in animals? Int. Rev. Neurobiol. 19 (1976) 1–49

133 Jannetta, P.J.: Observations on the etiology of trigeminal neuralgia, hemifacial spasm, acoustic nerve dysfunction and glossopharyngeal neuralgia. Definitive microsurgical treatment and results in 117 patients. Neurochirurgia 20 (1977) 145–154

134 Jannetta, P.J.: Hemifacial spasm. In: Samii, M., Jannetta, P.J. (Eds.): The cranial nerves. Berlin, Heidelberg, New York: Springer 1981 484–493

135 Jannetta, P.J., Bennett, M.H.: The pathophysiology of trigeminal neuralgia. In: Samii, M., Jannetta, P.J. (Eds.): The cranial nerves. Berlin, Heidelberg, New York: Springer 1981 312–315

136 Jansen, J., Brodal, A.: Das Kleinhirn. In: Möllendorff, W. von, Bargmann, W., Oksche, A., Vollrath, L. (Eds.): Handbuch der mikroskopischen Anatomie des Menschen. Vol. 4: Nervensystem, part 8. Berlin, Heidelberg, New York: Springer 1958

137 Janzen, R. (Ed.): Schmerzanalyse als Wegweiser zur Diagnose, 4th ed. Stuttgart: Thieme 1981

138 Jelgersma, G.: Atlas anatomicum cerebri humani. Amsterdam: Scheltema and Holkema N.V. 1931

139 Kahle, W., Leonhardt, H., Platzer, W.: Color atlas and textbook of human anatomy. Vol. 3: Nervous system and sensory organs. Stuttgart: Thieme 1978

140 Kandel, E.R., Schwartz, J.H. (Eds.): Principles of neural science. New York: Elsevier Science Publishing 1985

141 Kappert, A.: Neue nichtinvasive Untersuchungsmethoden bei zerebrovaskulärer Insuffizienz. Triangel 21 (1982) 1–11

142 Katada, K., Kanno, T., Sano, H., Shibata, T., Toda, T., Koga, S.: CT in evaluation of the circle of Willis. Neuroradiologie 16 (1978) 337–339

143 Kautzky, R., Zülch, K.J.: Neurologisch-neurochirurgische Röntgendiagnostik und andere Methoden zur Erkennung intrakranialer Erkrankungen. Berlin, Göttingen, Heidelberg: Springer 1955

144 Kautzky, R., Zülch, K.J., Wende, S., Tänzer, A.: Neuroradiologie auf neuropathologischer Grundlage. Berlin, Heidelberg, New York: Springer 1976

145 Kazner, E., Wende, S., Grumme, T., Lanksch, W., Stochdorph, O. (Eds.): Computertomographie intrakranieller Tumoren aus klinischer Sicht. Berlin, Heidelberg, New York: Springer 1981

146 Kerr, F.W.L.: Neuroanatomical substrates of nociception in the spinal cord. Pain 1 (1975) 325–356

147 Kertesz, A.: Aphasia and associated disorders; taxonomy, localization, and recovery. New York, London, Toronto: Grune and Stratton 1979

148 Keyserlingk, D. von, Lange, S.: Lagevariation von Hirnstrukturen im Bezugsystem der Computertomographie. Anat. Anz. 146 (1979) 245–255

149 Kieffer, S.A., Heitzman, E.R. (Eds.): An atlas of cross sectional anatomy. New York: Harper and Row 1979

150 Klingler, J.: Die makroskopische Anatomie der Ammonsformation. Denkschriften der Schweizerischen Naturforschenden Gesellschaft. Vol. 78, part 1. Zürich: Fretz 1948

151 Knudsen, P.A.: Ventriklernes storrelseforhold i anatomisk normale hjerner fra voksne mennesker. Odense: Andelsbogtrykkeriet 1958

152 Kömpf, D.: Supranukleäre und internukleäre Augenbewegungsstörungen. Fortschr. Neurol. Psychiat. 50 (1982) 143–164

153 Koritké, J.G., Sick, H.: Atlas of sectional human anatomy. Vol. 1: Head, neck, thorax. München: Urban und Schwarzenberg 1983

154 Kornhuber, H.H.: The vestibular system and the general motor system. In: Autrum, H., Jung, R., Loewenstein, W.R., Teuber, H.L. (Eds.): Handbook of sensory physiology. Vol. 6: Vestibular system, part 2. Berlin, Heidelberg, New York: Springer 1974 581–620

155 Kornhuber, H.H.: Physiologie und Pathophysiologie der corticalen und subcortikalen Bewegungssteuerung. In: Mertens, H.G., Przuntek, H. (Eds.): Verhandlungen der Deutschen Gesellschaft für Neurologie. Vol. 1: Pathologische Erregbarkeit des Nervensystems und ihre Behandlung. Berlin, Heidelberg, New York: Springer 1980 17–32

156 Krauland, W.: Über die Quellen des akuten und chronischen subduralen Hämatoms. In: Bargmann, W., Doerr, W. (Eds.): Zwanglose Abhandlungen aus dem Gebiet der normalen und pathologischen Anatomie, Heft 10. Stuttgart: Thieme 1961

157 Kretschmann, H.-J., Schleicher, A., Grottschreiber, J.-F., Kullmann, W.: The Yakovlev Collection. A pilot study of its suitability for the morphometric documentation of the human brain. J. neurol. Sci. 43 (1979) 111–126

158 Kretschmann, H.-J., Tafesse, U., Herrmann, A.: Different volume changes of cerebral cortex and white matter during histological preparation. Microscopica Acta 86 (1982) 13–24

159 Kretschmann, H.-J., Kammradt, G., Krauthausen, I., Sauer, B., Wingert, F.: Growth of the hippocampal formation in man. Bibliotheca anatomica Basel: Karger Vol. 28 (in press)

160 Kretschmer, H.: Neurotraumatologie. Stuttgart: Thieme 1978

161 Krieg, W.J.S.: Functional neuroanatomy. Bloomington/Ill.: Pantagraph Printing 1966

162 Krieg, W.J.S.: Architectonics of human cerebral fiber systems. Evanston/Ill.: Brain Books 1973

163 Künzle, H., Akert, K.: Efferent connections of cortical area 8 (frontal eye field) in Macaca fascicularis. A reinvestigation using the autoradiographic technique. J. comp. Neurol. 173 (1977) 147–164

164 Kuypers, H.G.J.M.: Corticobulbar connexions to the pons and lower brain-stem in man. Brain 81 (1958) 364–388

165 Kuypers, H.G.J.M.: Central cortical projections to motor and somatosensory cell groups. Brain 83 (1960) 161–184

166 Kuypers, H.G.J.M.: Anatomy of the descending pathways. In: Brooks, V.B. (Ed.): Handbook of physiology. Sec. 1: The nervous system, vol. 2: Motor Control, part 2. (American physiological society. ser.) Baltimore: Williams and Wilkins 1981 597–666

167 Lang, J.: Kopf: Gehirn- und Augenschädel. In: Lanz, T. von, Wachsmuth, W. (Eds.): Praktische Anatomie, Vol. 1, part 1B. Berlin, Heidelberg, New York: Springer 1979

168 Lang, J.: Clinical anatomy of the head. Berlin, Heidelberg, New York: Springer 1983

169 Lang, J., Stefanec, P., Breitenbach, W.: Über Form und Maße des Ventriculus tertius, von Sehbahnteilen und des N. oculomotorius. Neurochirurgica 26 (1983) 1–5

170 Lange, S., Grumme, Th., Weese, M.: Anatomie des Gehirns im Computertomogramm. Fortschr. Röntgenstr. 125 (1976) 421–427

171 Lange, S., Grumme, Th., Weese, M.: Zerebrale Computer-Tomographie. Berlin: Schering 1977

172 Langman, J.: Medical embryology. 4th ed. Baltimore: Williams and Wilkins 1981

173 Lassek, A.M.: The pyramidal tract. Springfield/Ill.: Thomas 1954

174 Last, R.J., Tompsett, D.H.: Casts of the cerebral ventricles. Brit. J. Surg. 40 (1953) 525–543

175 Lee, S.H., Rao, K.C.V.G.: Cranial computed tomography. New York: Mc Graw Hill 1983

176 Leischner, A.: Aphasien und Sprachentwicklungsstörungen. Klinik und Behandlung. Stuttgart: Thieme 1979

177 LeMay, M.: Asymmetries of the skull and handedness. J. neurol. Sci. 32 (1977) 243–253

178 Lemburg, P., Bretschneider, A., Storm, W.: Ultraschall zur Diagnostik morphologischer Hirnveränderungen bei Neugeborenen. Mschr. Kinderheilk. 129 (1981) 190–199

179 Leonhardt, H.: Ependym und circumventriculäre Organe. In: Möllendorff, W. von, Bargmann, W., Oksche, A., Vollrath, L. (Eds.): Handbuch der mikroskopischen Anatomie des Menschen. Vol. 4: Nervensystem, part 10. Berlin, Heidelberg, New York: Springer 1980 177–666

180 Lindenberg, R.: Die Gefäßversorgung und ihre Bedeutung für Art und Ort von kreislaufbedingten Gewebsschäden und Gefäßprozessen. In: Lubarsch, O., Henke, F., Rössle, R., Uehlinger, E. (Eds.): Handbuch der speziellen pathologischen Anatomie und Histologie. Vol. 13: Nervensystem, part 1/B. Berlin, Heidelberg, New York: Springer 1957 1071–1164

181 Ludwig, E., Klingler, J.: Atlas cerebri humani. Basel: Karger 1956

182 Lukes, St.A., Crooks, L.E., Aminoff, M.J., Kaufman, L., Panitch, H.S., Mills, C., Norman, D.: Nuclear magnetic resonance imaging in multiple sclerosis. Ann. Neurol. 13 (1983) 592–601

183 Maat, G.J.R., Vielvoye, G.J., Tinkelenberg, J.: An anatomical aid for the evaluation of computed tomography scans. Beetsterzwaag: Mefar 1981

184 Mancuso, A.: Computed tomography of head and neck. Baltimore: Williams and Wilkins 1982

185 Martin, W.R.W., Beckman, J.H., Calne, D.B., Adam, M.J., Harrop, R., Rogers, J.G., Ruth, T.J., Sayre, C.I., Pate, B.D.: Cerebral glucose metabolism in Parkinson's disease. Can. J. Neurol. Sci. 11 (1984) 169–173

186 McGeer, P.L., Eccles, J.C., McGeer, E.G.: Molecular neurobiology of the mammalian brain. New York, London: Plenum 1978

187 McGrath, Ph., Mills, P.: Atlas of sectional anatomy. Head, neck, and trunk. Basel: Karger 1984

188 Matsui, T., Hirano, A.: An atlas of the human brain for computerized tomography. Stuttgart, New York: Fischer 1978

189 Matsui, T., Kawamoto, K., Iwata, M., Kurent, J.E., Imai, T., Ohsugi, T., Hirano, A.: Anatomical and pathological study of the brain by CT scanner. 1: Anatomical study of normal brain. Comput. Tomogr. 1 (1977) 3–43

190 Mawad, M.E., Silver, A.J., Hilal, S.K., Ganti, S.R.: Computed tomography of the brain stem with intrathecal metrizamide. Part I: The normal brain stem. Amer. J. Roentgenol. 140 (1983) 553–563

191 Meese, W., Kluge, W., Grumme, T., Hopfenmüller, W.: CT evaluation of the CSF spaces of healthy persons. Neuroradiology 19 (1980) 131–136

192 Meschan, I.: Synopsis of radiologic anatomy with computed tomography. Philadelphia, London, Toronto: Saunders 1980

193 Moore, R.Y., Bloom, F.E.: Central catecholamine neuron systems: Anatomy and physiology of the dopamine systems. Ann. Rev. Neurosci. 1 (1978) 129–169

194 Moore, R.Y., Bloom, F.E.: Central catecholamine neuron systems: Anatomy and physiology of the norepinephrine and epinephrine systems. Ann. Rev. Neurosci. 2 (1979) 113–168

195 Morgane, P.J., Panksepp, J. (Eds): Handbook of the hypothalamus. Vol. 1: Anatomy of the hypothalamus. New York: Dekker 1979

196 Mumenthaler, M.: Neurologische Differentialdiagnostik. Stuttgart: Thieme 1983

197 Mumenthaler, M.: Neurology. Stuttgart, New York: Thieme-Stratton 1983

198 Mundinger, F., Birg, W.: Stereotactic brain surgery with the aid of computed tomography (CT-stereotaxy). Advanc. Neurosurg. 10 (1982) 17–24

199 Nadjmi, M., Piepgras, U., Vogelsang, H.: Kranielle Computertomographie. Stuttgart, New York: Thieme 1981

200 Nadjmi, M., Ratzka, M., Wodarz, R., Glötzner, F.L.: Bedeutung der Computertomographie für die Neuroradiologie. Röntgen-Berichte 6 (1977) 258–293

201 Naidich, T.P., Leeds, N.E., Kricheff, I.I., Pudlowski, R.M., Naidich, J.B., Zimmerman, R.D.: The tentorium in axial section. Radiology 123 (1977) 631–648

202 Naidich, T.P., Pudlowski, R.M., Leeds, N.E., Naidich, J.B., Chisolm, A.J., Rifkin, M.D.: The normal contrast-enhanced computed axial tomogram of the brain. J. Comput. assist. Tomogr. 1 (1977) 16–29

203 Nauta, W.J.H., Haymaker, W.: Hypothalamic nuclei and fiber connections. In: Haymaker, W., Anderson, E., Nauta, W.J.H. (Eds.): The hypothalamus. Springfield/Ill.: Thomas 1969 136–209

204 New, P.F.J., Scott, W.R.: Computed tomography of the brain and orbit. Baltimore: Williams and Wilkins 1975

205 Newton, Th.H., Potts, D.G. (Eds.): Radiology of the skull and brain. Technical aspects of computed tomography. Vol. 5. St. Louis, Toronto, London: Mosby 1981

206 Nieuwenhuys, R., Voogd, J., Huijzen, C. van: The human central nervous system. A synopsis and atlas. 2nd ed. Berlin, Heidelberg, New York: Springer 1981

207 Noback, C.R., Demarest, R.J.: The human nervous system. Basic principles of neurobiology. 3rd ed. New York: McGraw-Hill 1980

208 Nobin, A., Björklund, A.: Topography of the monoamine neuron systems in the human brain as revealed in fetuses. Acta physiol. scand., Suppl. 388 (1973) 1–40

209 Nygrèn, L.-G., Olson, L.: A new major projection from locus coeruleus: The main source of noradrenergic nerve terminals in the ventral and dorsal columns of the spinal cord. Brain Res. 132 (1977) 85–93

210 Ojemann, G.A.: The intrahemispheric organization of human language, derived with electrical stimulation techniques. Trends in Neuroscience 6 (1983) 184–189

211 Oldendorf, W.H.: Isolated flying spot detection of radiodensity discontinuities-displaying the internal structural pattern of a complex object. IRE Trans. biomed. electr. (N.Y.) 8 (1961) 68–72

212 Olszewski, J.: The thalamus of the macaca mulatta. An atlas for use with stereotaxic instruments. Basel, New York: Karger 1952

213 Olszewski, J., Baxter, D.: Cytoarchitecture of the human brain stem. Basel, New York: Karger 1982

214 Osborn, A.G.: The medial tentorium and incisura: normal and pathological anatomy. Neuroradiology 13 (1977) 109–113

215 Palay, S.L., Chan-Palay, V.: Cerebellar cortex. Cytology and organization. Berlin, Heidelberg, New York: Springer 1974

216 Panofsky, W., Staemmler, M.: Untersuchungen über Hirngewicht und Schädelkapazität nach der Reichardtschen Methode. Frankfurt. Z. Path. 26 (1922) 519–549

217 Papeschi, R.: Dopamine, extrapyramidal system, and psychomotor function. Psychiat. Neurol. Neurochir. (Amst.) 75 (1972) 13–48

218 Partain, C.L., James, A.E., Rollo, F.D., Price, R.R. (Eds.): Nuclear magnetic resonance (NMR) imaging. Philadelphia: Saunders 1983

219 Patten, J.: Neurological differential diagnosis. Berlin, Heidelberg, New York: Springer 1982

220 Penfield, W., Rasmussen, T.: The cerebral cortex of man. A clinical study of localization of function. New York: Macmillan 1950

221 Penfield, W., Welch, K.: The supplementary motor area of the cerebral cortex. A clinical and experimental study. Arch. Neurol. Psychiat. (Chic.) 66 (1951) 289–317

222 Perenin, M.T., Jeannerod, M.: Subcortical vision in man. Trends in Neuroscience 2 (1979) 204–207

223 Pernkopf, E.: Atlas of topographical and applied human anatomy. Vol. 1: Head and neck. München, Wien, Baltimore: Urban und Schwarzenberg 1980

224 Peters, A., Palay, S.L., Webster, H.F. de: The fine structure of the nervous system: The neurons and supporting cells. Philadelphia, London, Toronto: Saunders 1976

225 Petersilka, E., Pfeiler, M.: Zur Technik der Computertomographie. Röntgen-Berichte 6 (1977) 233–257

226 Piepgras, U.: Neuroradiologie. Stuttgart, New York: Thieme 1977

227 Pigadas, A., Thompson, J.R., Grube, G.L.: Normal infant brain anatomy: Correlated real-time sonograms and brain specimens. Amer. J. Roentgenol. 137 (1981) 815–820

228 Platzer, W.: Atlas of Topographical Anatomy. Stuttgart: Thieme 1985

229 Plum, F., Posner, J.B.: The diagnosis of stupor and coma. 2nd ed. Contemporary Neurology Series. Philadelphia: Davis 1978

230 Poeck, K.: Neurologie. Berlin, Heidelberg, New York: Springer 1982

231 Poeck, K. (Ed.): Klinische Neuropsychologie. Stuttgart, New York: Thieme 1982

232 Pompeiano, O.: Reticular formation. In: Autrum, H., Jung, R., Loewenstein, W.R., Teuber, H. (Eds.): Handbook of sensory physiology. Vol. 2: Somatosensory system. Berlin, Heidelberg, New York: Springer 1973 381–488

233 Pöppel, E., Held, R., Dowling, J.E.: Neural mechanisms in visual perception. Neurosci. Res. Program Bull. 15 (1977) 313–319, 323–353

234 Quaknine, G.E.: Microsurgical anatomy of the arterial loops in the ponto-cerebellar angle and the internal acoustic meatus. In: Samii, M., Jannetta, P.J. (Eds.): The cranial nerves. Berlin, Heidelberg, New York: Springer 1981 378–390

235 Radü, E.W., Kendall, B.E., Moseley, I.F.: Computertomographie des Kopfes. Stuttgart, New York: Thieme 1980

236 Raichle, M.E., Hartman, B.K., Eichling, J.O., Sharpe, L.G.: Central noradrenergic regulation of cerebral blood flow and vascular permeability. Proc. nat. Acad. Sci. (Wash.) 72 (1975) 3726–3730

237 Ramsey, R.G.: Neuroradiology with computed tomography. Philadelphia, London: Saunders 1981

238 Ramsey, R.G.: Diagnostic radiology of the brain: CT, DSA, NMR. 2nd ed. In: Advanced exercises in diagnostic radiology. Vol. 9. Philadelphia, London: Saunders 1984

239 Rath, M., Lissner, J.: Computertomographie: Indikationen und derzeitige Wertigkeit. Med. Klin. 77 (1982) 538–545

240 Reisner, K., Gosepath, J.: Craniotomography. An atlas and guide. Stuttgart, New York: Thieme-Stratton 1977

241 Reisner, Th.: Die klinische Bedeutung der kranialen Computertomographie in der Neuropädiatrie. Wien. klin. Wschr. 93, Suppl. 130 (1981) 1–33

242 Reisner, Th., Zeiler, K., Strobl, G.: Quantitative Erfassung der Seitenventrikelbreite im CT – Vergleichswerte einer Normalpopulation. Fortschr. Neurol. Psychiat. 48 (1980) 168–174

243 Retzius, G.: Das Menschenhirn. Studien in der makroskopischen Morphologie. Vol. I. Stockholm: Norstedt 1896

244 Reynolds, A.F., Harris, A.B., Ojemann, G.A., Turner, P.T.: Aphasia and left thalamic hemorrhage. J. Neurosurg. 48 (1978) 570–574

245 Riley, H.A.: An Atlas of the basal ganglia, brain stem, and spinal cord. New York: Hafner 1960

246 Ring, A., Waddington, M.M.: Roentgenographic anatomy of the pericallosal arteries. Amer. J. Roentgenol. 104 (1968) 109–118

247 Robertson, E.G.: Pneumoencephalography. Springfield/Ill.: Thomas 1967

248 Robertson, L.T., Dow, R.S.: Anatomy of the cerebellum. In: Schaltenbrand, G., Walker, A.E. (Eds.): Stereotaxy of the human brain, 2nd ed. Stuttgart, New York: Thieme 1982 60–70

249 Röthig, W.: Korrelationen zwischen Gesamthirn- und Kleinhirngewicht des Menschen im Laufe der Ontogenese. J. Hirnforsch. 15 (1974) 203–209

250 Rosene, D.L., Hoesen, G.W. van: Hippocampal efferents reach wide-spread areas of cerebral cortex and amygdala in the rhesus monkey. Science 198 (1977) 315–317

251 Ross, E.D.: Localization of the pyramidal tract in the internal capsule by whole brain dissection. Neurology 30 (1980) 59–64

252 Roth, K.: NMR-Tomographie und -Spektroskopie in der Medizin. Berlin, Heidelberg, New York: Springer 1984

253 Rottenberg, D.A., Talman, W., Chernik, N.L.: Letter: Location of pyramidal tract questioned. Neurology 26 (1976) 291–292

254 Rowland, L.P.: Clinical syndromes of the brain stem. In: Kandel, E.R., Schwartz, J.H. (Eds.): Principles of neural science. New York: Elsevier Science Publishing 1983 419–430

255 Sabattini, L.: Evaluation and measurement of the normal ventricular and subarachnoid spaces by CT. Neuroradiology 23 (1982) 1–5

256 Sachsenweger, R.: Neuroophthalmologie, 3rd ed. Stuttgart: Thieme 1982

257 Salamon, G., Huang, Y.P.: Radiologic anatomy of the brain. Berlin, Heidelberg, New York: Springer 1976

258 Salamon, G., Huang, Y.P.: Computed tomography of the brain. Berlin, Heidelberg, New York: Springer 1980

259 Salamon, G., Lecaque, G., Hall, K., Corbaz, J.M.: C.A.T. scanning: correlations with vascular and topographical anatomy. In: Boulay, G.H. du, Moseley, I.F. (Eds.): Computerised axial tomography in clinical practice. Berlin, Heidelberg, New York: Springer 1977 17–23

260 Salvolini, U., Cabanis, E.A., Rodallec, A., Menichelli, F., Pasquini, U., Iba-Zizen, M.T.: Computed tomography of the optic nerve. Part I: Normal results. J. Comput. assist. Tomogr. 2 (1978) 141–149

261 Samii, M., Jannetta, P.J. (Eds.): The cranial nerves. Berlin, Heidelberg, New York: Springer 1981

262 Sanides, F.: Representation in the cerebral cortex and its areal lamination patterns. In: Bourne, G.H. (Ed.): The structure and function of nervous tissue. New York, London: Academic Press 1972 329–453

263 Sarkisoff, S.A., Filimonoff, I.N.: Atlas du cerveau de l'homme et des animaux. Moscou 1937

264 Schaltenbrand, G., Bailey, P.: Einführung in die stereotaktischen Operationen mit einem Atlas des menschlichen Gehirns. Stuttgart: Thieme 1959

265 Schaltenbrand, G., Wahren, W.: Atlas for stereotaxy of the human brain, 2nd ed. Stuttgart, New York: Thieme 1977

266 Schaltenbrand, G., Walker, A.E. (Eds.): Stereotaxy of the human brain. Anatomical, physiological and clinical applications, 2nd ed. Stuttgart: Thieme 1982

267 Scheid, W.: Lehrbuch der Neurologie, 5th ed. Stuttgart: Thieme 1983

268 Scheuerlein, H.: Single-Photon-Emissionstomographie. Röntgenstrahlen 48 (1982) 24–27

269 Schiebler, T.H., Schmidt, W. (Eds.): Lehrbuch der gesamten Anatomie des Menschen. 3rd ed. Berlin: Springer 1983

270 Schiffter, R.: Die klinische Phänomenologie der supra- und internukleären Augenmuskellähmungen. Akt. Neurol. 1 (1974) 61–67

271 Schmidt, H.-M.: Über Größe, Form und Lage von Bulbus und Tractus olfactorius des Menschen. Gegenbaurs morph. Jb. (Lpzg.) 119 (1973) 227–237

272 Schnitzlein, H.N., Murtagh, F.R.: Imaging anatomy of the head and spine. Baltimore, Munich: Urban und Schwarzenberg 1985

273 Schultze, W.H.: Über Messungen und Untersuchungen des Liquor cerebrospinalis an der Leiche. In: Schmidt, M.B., Berblinger, W. (Eds.): Centralblatt für allgemeine Pathologie und pathologische Anatomie. Suppl. of Vol. 33. Jena: Fischer 1923 291–296

274 Schumacher, R.: Ultraschalluntersuchungen des Hirnschädels von Neugeborenen und Säuglingen mit einem neuen Schallkopf. Electromedica 50 (1982) 70–76

275 Schuy, S., Leitgeb, N.: Übersichtsvortrag Grenzen und Möglichkeiten der Ultraschalldiagnostik. Biomed. Technik 26 (1981) 49–54

276 Seeger, W.: Atlas of topographical anatomy of the brain and surrounding structures for neurosurgeons, neuroradiologists, and neuropathologists. Wien, New York: Springer 1978

277 Shipps, F.C.: Atlas of brain anatomy for CT scans using EMI terminology. Springfield/Ill.: Thomas 1977

278 Sidman, R.L., Rakic, P.: Development of the human central nervous system. In: Haymaker, W., Adams, R.D. (Eds.): Histology and histopathology of the nervous system. Vol. 1. Springfield/Ill.: Thomas 1982 3–145

279 Singer, M., Yakovlev, P.I.: The human brain in sagittal section. Springfield/Ill.: Thomas 1964

280 Singer, W.: Control of thalamic transmission by corticofugal and ascending reticular pathways in the visual system. Physiol. Rev. 57 (1977) 386–420

281 Smith, C.G., Richardson, W.F.G.: The course and distribution of the arteries supplying the visual (striate) cortex. Amer. J. Ophthal. 61 (1966) 1391–1396

282 Smith, R.L.: Axonal projections and connections of the principal sensory trigeminal nucleus in the monkey. J. comp. Neurol. 163 (1975) 347–376

283 Sobotta, J., Ferner, H., Staubesand, J. (Eds.): Atlas of human anatomy. With nomenclature in English. 10th ed. Vol. 1: Head, neck, upper extremities. Baltimore, Munich: Urban und Schwarzenberg 1983

284 Spatz, H.: Anatomie des Mittelhirns. In: Bumke, O., Foerster, O. (Eds.): Handbuch der Neurologie. Vol. I: Allgemeine Neurologie. Berlin: Springer 1935 474–540

285 Starck, D.: Die Evolution des Säugetier-Gehirns. Wiesbaden: Steiner 1962

286 Starck, D.: Embryologie, 3rd ed. Stuttgart: Thieme 1975

287 Starck, D.: Vergleichende Anatomie der Wirbeltiere. Vol. III. Berlin, Heidelberg, New York: Springer 1982

288 Staudt, F., Henne, K., Heinzerling, J.: Zweidimensionale Echoenzephalographie bei Neugeborenen und Säuglingen mit dem Sonodiagnost R 2000. Röntgenstrahlen 48 (1982) 18–23

289 Stephan, H.: Allocortex. In: Möllendorff, W. von, Bargmann, W., Oksche, A., Vollrath, L. (Eds.): Handbuch der mikroskopischen Anatomie des Menschen. Vol. IV: Nervensystem, part 9. Berlin, Heidelberg, New York: Springer 1975

290 Stephan, H., Andy, O.J.: Anatomy of the limbic system. In: Schaltenbrand, G., Walker, A.E. (Eds.): Stereotaxy of the

human brain, 2nd ed. Stuttgart, New York: Thieme 1982 269–292

291 Stokely, E.M., Sveinsdottir, E., Lassen, N.A., Rommer, P.: A single photon dynamic computer assisted tomograph (DCAT) for imaging brain function in multiple cross sections. J. Comput. assist. Tomogr. 4 (1980) 230–240

292 Strassburg, H.-M., Weber, S., Sauer, M.: Diagnosing hydrocephalus in infants by ultrasound sector scanning through the open fontanelles. A study comparing ultrasound-sonography and cat-scan. Neuropediatrics 12 (1981) 254–266

293 Svendsen, P., Duru, O.: Visibility of the temporal horns on computed tomography. Neuroradiology 21 (1981) 139–144

294 Swanson, L.W.: The locus coeruleus: a cytoarchitectonic, Golgi, and immunohistochemical study in the albino rat. Brain Res. 110 (1976) 39–56

295 Székely, G.: Order and plasticity in the nervous system. Trends in Neuroscience 2 (1979) 245–248

296 Szikla, G., Bouvier, G., Hori, T., Petrov, V.: Angiography of the human brain cortex. Berlin, Heidelberg, New York: Springer 1977

297 Takahashi, S. (Ed.): Illustrated computer tomography. Berlin, Heidelberg, New York: Springer 1983

298 Takase, M., Tokunaga, A., Otani, K., Horie, T.: Atlas of the human brain for computed tomography based on the glabella-inion-line. Neuroradiology 14 (1977) 73–79

299 Thompson, J.R., Hasso, A.N.: Correlative sectional anatomy of the head and neck. St. Louis, Toronto, London: Mosby 1980

300 Töndury, G.: Angewandte und topographische Anatomie, 5th ed. Stuttgart: Thieme 1981

301 Toole, J.F., Patel, A.N.: Zerebro-vaskuläre Störungen. Berlin, Heidelberg, New York: Springer 1980

302 Unsöld, R., Ostertag, C.B., Groot, J. de, Newton, T.H.: Computer reformations of the brain and skull base. Berlin, Heidelberg, New York: Springer 1982

303 Unterharnscheidt, F., Jachnik, D., Gött, H.: Der Balkenmangel. Berlin, Heidelberg, New York: Springer 1968

304 Valk, J.: Computed tomography and cerebral infarctions. New York: Raven 1980

305 Vogt, C., Vogt, O.: Sitz und Wesen der Krankheiten im Lichte der topistischen Hirnforschung und des Variierens der Tiere. J. Psychol. Neurol. (Lpzg.) 47 (1937) 237–457

306 Vogt, U.: Zur Bedeutung obturierender Prozesse in zuführenden Hirngefäßen. Stuttgart: Thieme 1973

307 Volpe, J.J.: Anterior fontanel: Window to the neonatal brain. J. Pediatrics 100 (1982) 395–398

308 Voogd, J.: The cerebellum of the cat. Assen: Van Gorcum 1964

309 Wackenheim, A., Jeanmart, L., Baert, A.L.: Craniocerebral computer tomography. Vol. 1. Berlin, Heidelberg, New York: Springer 1980

310 Waddington, M.M.: Atlas of cerebral angiography with anatomic correlations. Boston: Little and Brown 1974

311 Walker, A.E.: The primate thalamus. Chicago: University Press 1966

312 Walker, A.E.: Normal and pathological physiology of the thalamus. In: Schaltenbrand, G., Walker, A.E. (Eds.): Stereotaxy of the human brain, 2nd ed. Stuttgart, New York: Thieme 1982 181–217

313 Wegener, O.H.: Whole body computerized tomography. Basel, New York: Karger 1983

314 Weinstein, M.A., Modic, M.T., Risius, B., Duchesneau, P.M., Berlin, A.J.: Visualization of the arteries, veins, and nerves of the orbit by sector computed tomography. Radiology 138 (1981) 83–87

315 Wende, S., Thelen, M.: Kernspintomographie in der Medizin. Berlin, Heidelberg, New York: Springer 1983

316 Wessely, W.: Biometrische Analyse der Frischvolumina des Rhombencephalon, des Cerebellum und der Ventrikel von 31 adulten menschlichen Gehirnen. J. Hirnforsch. 12 (1970) 11–28

317 Wiesendanger, M.: The pyramidal tract recent investigations on its morphology and function. Ergebn. Physiol. 61 (1969) 72–136

318 Williams, P.L., Warwick, R.: Gray's anatomy. 36th ed. Edingburgh: Churchill Livingstone 1980

319 Willis, W.D., Grossman, R.G.: Medical neurobiology. Neuroanatomical and neurophysiological principles basic to clinical neuroscience. St. Louis: Mosby 1977

320 Wolf, G.: Epiphysen- und Plexusverkalkungen in der Computertomographie. Med. Dissertation Hannover Medical School 1980

321 Wood, J.H.: Neurobiology of cerebrospinal fluid. New York: Plenum 1980

322 Yamamoto, Y., Satoh, T., Asari, S., Sadamoto, K.: Normal anatomy of cerebral vessels by computed angiotomography in the axial transverse plane. J. Comput. assist. Tomogr. 6 (1982) 865–873

323 Yamamoto, Y., Satoh, T., Asari, S., Sadamoto, K.: Normal anatomy of cerebral vessels by computed angiotomography in the coronal, Towne, and semisagittal planes. J. Comput. assist. Tomogr. 6 (1982) 1049–1057

324 Yamamoto, Y., Satoh, T., Sakurai, M., Asari, S., Sadamoto, K.: Minimum dose contrast bolus in computed angiotomography of the brain. J. Comput. assist. Tomogr. 6 (1982) 575–585

325 Yasargil, M.G.: Microneurosurgery. Vol. 1. Stuttgart, New York: Thieme-Stratton 1984

326 Young, I.R., Bailes, D.R., Burl, M., Collins, A.G., Smith, D.T., McDonnell, M.J., Orr, J.S., Banks, L.M., Bydder, G.M., Greenspan, R.H., Steiner, R.E.: Initial clinical evaluation of a whole body nuclear magnetic resonance (NMR) tomograph. J. Comput. assist. Tomogr. 6 (1982) 1–18

327 Zeitler, E., Schittenhelm, R.: Die Kernspintomographie und ihre klinischen Anwendungsmöglichkeiten. Electromedica 49 (1981) 134–143

328 Zeumer, H., Hacke, W., Hartwich, P.: A quantitative approach to measuring the cerebrospinal fluid space. Neuroradiology 22 (1982) 193–197

329 Zilles, K.: Determination und Plastizität in der prä- und postnatalen Entwicklung des Gehirns. Z. mikr.-anat. Forsch. 93 (1979) 763–779

330 Zonneveld, F.W.: Computer Tomographie. Eindhoven/Netherlands: Philips Medical Systems 1981

331 Zülch, K.J., Creutzfeldt, O.D., Galbraith, G.C. (Eds.): Cerebral localization. New York, Heidelberg, Berlin: Springer 1975

332 Zuleger, S., Staubesand, J.: Schnittbilder des Zentralnervensystems. München, Wien, Baltimore: Urban und Schwarzenberg 1976

6 Index for Text and Illustrations

Plain numbers refer to pages. Numbers preceded by the letter F refer to figures. On the inside front cover the reader finds a list giving the page numbers of each illustration.

Example: The angular gyrus F 4.11 can be found on page 16 in Figure 4 and is indicated by number 11.